FAMILY

FIRST AID

AND EMERGENCY HANDBOOK

Contents

Contents

FAMILY

FIRST AID

AND EMERGENCY HANDBOOK

Dr Andrew Stanway MB MRCP

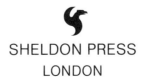

SHELDON PRESS

LONDON

Designed and produced for the Boots Company Limited
by The Rainbird Publishing Group Limited,
40 Park Street,
London W1Y 4DE

First published in paperback
in Great Britain in 1984
by Sheldon Press, SPCK
Marylebone Road, London
NW1 4DU

Text: © Andrew Stanway MB, MRCP, 1980

Design and illustration: Linda Rogers Associates

Set, printed and bound by
Mackays of Chatham Ltd

British Library Cataloguing in Publication Data

Stanway, Andrew
    Family first aid.—(Overcoming common problems)
    1. First aid in illness and injury
    I. Title   II. Series
    616.02′52   RC87

    ISBN 0–85969–413–5

Acknowledgements

I should like to thank the many individuals and organisations that have
given me so much help in the preparation of this book but in particular
the following:
British Gas
The Chief Fire Officer of Surrey
Derek Carter
The Flowers and Plants Council
The Health Education Council
MIND
The Royal Society for the Prevention of Accidents
The Sports Medicine Clinic, St James's Hospital, Leeds
Cyril Young MSc; MRCOG
Many of the self help organisations whose names and addresses
appear on pages 112 and 113. And especially Dr Roger Snook,
Consultant in Accident and Emergency Medicine at The Royal United
Hospital, Bath, who read through the manuscript and offered such
valuable advice in the light of his considerable experience in this field.

Useful telephone numbers

General Practitioner: _____

Local Hospital: _565656 frenchay_

Health Visitor: _____

Local Police Station: _____

* Chemist: _____

Community Health Council: _____

Samaritans: _____

Father's work no.: _____

Mother's work no.: _560436_

St John Ambulance: _____

Red Cross: _____

St Andrew's: _____

Other useful numbers: _____

* You can always find out which chemist shop is open out of hours by looking on the door of any local chemist, by consulting the list in your local police station, or by looking in the local paper.

Calling an ambulance

1 Dial Emergency

2 When the operator answers he will ask for your telephone number so that he can ring you back should you be cut off.

3 When asked whether you want Fire, Police or Ambulance, say 'ambulance'.

4 When you get through to the ambulance officer, tell him briefly what the emergency is.

5 Give directions to guide the ambulance to your home, especially if it is difficult to find, has a name and no number etc. It is helpful to go out to the nearest road intersection to meet the ambulance if you live in an out of the way place they might not find easily.

6 When the ambulance arrives, describe what has happened.

7 Get someone to look after the children or other relatives while you go off. If your child is the patient, always try to go with him.

8 Take your money with you and your front door key. Ambulances are under no obligation to deliver you back home so you'll need money for a taxi or bus.

Introduction

This is not a book of first aid in the popular sense of the phrase. Such books are usually written by experts in the management of accidents and leave the average householder feeling rather helpless because he can't quickly remember how to apply the right bandage correctly or master the specialised lifts and splints so beloved of professional first aiders. Most first aid books are aimed primarily at those studying the subject in groups and as such are not suitable for use in the home. They cover anatomy and physiology and are written in long, wordy passages that are difficult, if not impossible, to decipher in a domestic emergency.

In writing this book I have taken great pains to make the material easy to read, easy to understand and easy to carry out. This then is not a first aid book so much as a domestic emergency book that anyone who can read can use in real life situations. Most of it is common sense but even common sense can be misapplied and so lead to tragedy. For this reason I've tried to explain most of the common errors that people make.

Even though it's not a typical first aid book, most of the book does, however, give advice on 'first' as opposed to 'second' aid, although in many cases the second aid may never be necessary. This is desirable because so many people find that the time and trouble involved in seeking medical or hospital care is too great, especially when they're dealing with something relatively simple. The trouble is in knowing when something is simple. Throughout the book I've tried to point out when medical help ('second aid') is required because most people, quite understandably, don't want to take responsibility for things they feel unable to cope with easily. Nor should they do so.

However, it's not only accidents that concern us at home. What often worries us more is the heart attack that Dad had, the time little Johnny swallowed the bleach, or Aunt Freda's epileptic fits. Mum has a terrible time with her cystitis and Grandad stopped passing his water the other day. All of these things may constitute serious domestic emergencies and most of us are at a loss to know what to do in such cases. This book tells you.

Please turn to page 6 to read the Safety at home section; learn how to act should someone's heart stop or should he stop breathing (see pages 24 and 20 respectively); briefly familiarise yourself with the layout of the rest of the book and then put it away somewhere accessible and ensure that everyone knows where it is in an emergency. There can't be many books of which the author says 'I hope you don't need it' but this is certainly one.

ANDREW STANWAY MB; MRCP

NOTE
Throughout the book, illustrations are accompanied by a letter (or number) linked to the text.

Safety at home

Although many learned researchers talk about the psychodynamics of accidents everywhere and especially at home, there is little doubt that most accidents are caused through carelessness and thoughtlessness. Over 1½ million people are involved in accidents in their homes every year, a figure which considerably exceeds the far more widely publicised figure for road accidents in numbers if not in severity. Accidents at home account for 1 in 24 of all deaths or 37% of all accidental deaths in Great Britain. This might not sound much but it represents over 6,500 people dying in any one year. The very old and the very young are especially at risk from domestic hazards—the young because they are learning and the old because they are forgetting.

Most accidents occur in the kitchen (16%) and living room (16%) with the seemingly more dangerous garden next (11%). In the very young, falls, burns and scalds, fires, suffocation and poisoning head the list of dangers whereas older children suffer cuts, bruises and broken bones. Old people may accidentally take too many drugs. They may also fall more as their senses dull and this leads to an increase in cuts and burns. Seventy five per cent of all injuries needing hospital treatment are cuts and bruises, sprains, fractures, dislocations, burns and scalds.

Prevention often simply involves careful planning of your living to reduce the risk of accidents but however careful you are there are always special hazards encountered with fire, electricity, gas and water.

Fire can often be prevented. The Home Office booklet *Danger from Fire* is free to every household and is well worth reading. It's aimed at prevention and is available from some council offices, local Fire Prevention Departments and County Fire Brigade HQs.

Electricity and gas in the house should be treated with respect. Always consult experts if in doubt. Many domestic fires start because of unsafe wiring, plugs and appliances. The Electricity Council has produced a booklet *Safety in the Home* which is available from electricity showrooms or the Council itself. Another very good booklet is *Electricity for Everyday Living*. This is available from EAW (Publications Dept. Ltd), 25 Foubert's Place, London W1V 2AL, price 75p. The British Gas Corporation publishes the useful booklet *Help Yourself to Gas Safety*, available from your gas showroom.

For more information about safety at home, write to RoSPA and ask for the information you require. *Safe as Houses* is a particularly useful booklet and may be obtained for 65p per copy from RoSPA. (For address see page 113).

Thinking about safety can't start too young. If you have little children you have moral and certain legal responsibilities to protect them from danger. Remember too that a child under the age of 16 cannot be held responsible for the safety and well being of himself or for another child under 16—you as the adult are responsible. Get your children to respect danger, especially fire, gas, electricity and water and encourage them to think of the safety of others as soon as they are old enough. It's never too soon to start planning for safety.

Make today your starting point to go around the house, check off the points on the next twelve pages and **do something** about them if necessary. That ten minutes could be the most profitable you're likely to spend for some time.

6 Safety at home

Kitchen

1. Have cupboards that can easily be reached without having to stand on chairs or steps.
2. Turn handles of saucepans sideways.
3. Keep poisons, cleaning fluids and disinfectants high up and preferably locked.
4. Don't prise open cans with fingers.
5. Never leave fat heating in a pan on the cooker unattended.
6. Wipe up spills at once.
7. Don't highly polish floors.
8. Put all sharp things in drawers.
9. Check safety of plugs and wiring on domestic appliances.
10. Don't overload sockets.
11. Use a brush and dustpan to sweep up broken glass or china.
12. Have a fire extinguisher or fire blanket handy and learn how to use it.
13. Never put water on a fat fire—put a lid on the pan or cover with a fire blanket.
14. Teach children to respect kitchen machinery.
15. Have a first aid kit handy.
16. Never leave a flex overhanging from an electric kettle.

3 Don't

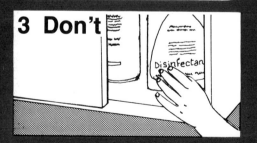

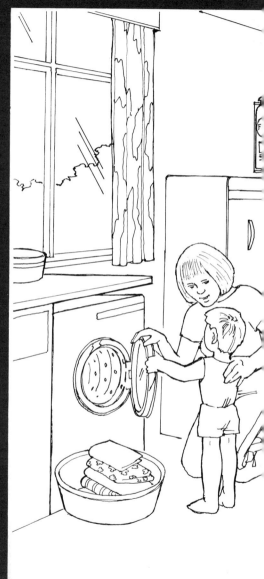

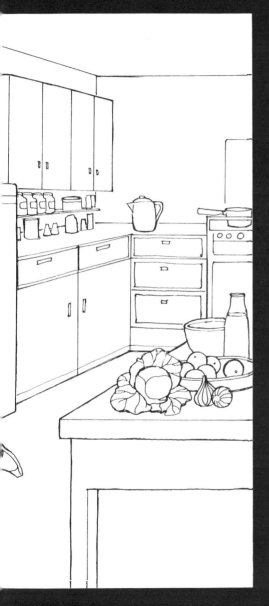

4 Don't

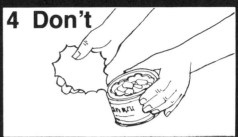

8 Don't

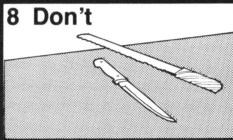

10 Don't

16 Don't

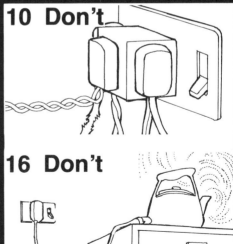

Bathroom

1 Keep all drugs and medicines out of children's reach, preferably in a special cupboard that locks.

2 Place medicine cupboard high on the wall so that children can't reach it.

3 Flush all old medicines and those without labels down the lavatory.

4 Ask the Gas Board to service the water heater yearly.

5 Choose non-slip flooring.

6 Have non-slip backing to bathroom mat.

7 Use a non-slip mat in the bath for the young and old.

8 Run cold water before hot when filling bath.

9 Ban portable mains-operated electric appliances from the bathroom.

10 The heater should be high up on the wall or ceiling but not over the bath.

11 Have a pull cord for light switch.

12 Have a proper razor socket only—no other power outlets.

13 Keep razors well out of children's reach.

14 Never block ventilation holes.

15 Never leave children alone in the bath.

5 Don't

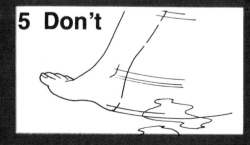

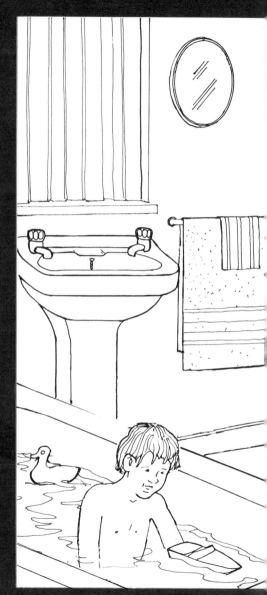

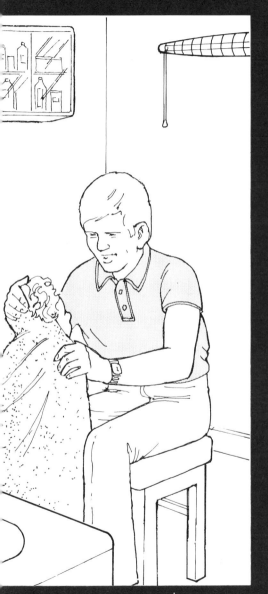

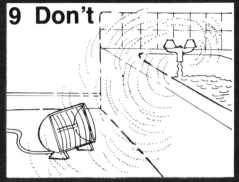

9 Don't

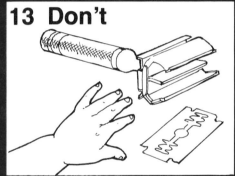

13 Don't

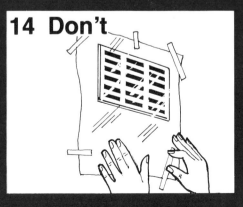

14 Don't

Shed, garage and workshop

1 Use the right tool—don't make do.

2 Use ramps for cars, not piles of bricks.

3 Keep garden tools hanging safely on walls.

4 Keep weedkiller and other chemicals high up and out of reach. **Never** use domestic containers (eg lemonade bottles) for weedkiller.

5 Check child's bike for safety at least twice a year.

6 Wear safety goggles or glasses when sanding or grinding.

7 Wear a mask when spraying and ventilate the area.

8 Work in a good light.

9 Petrol must be kept in metal cans only (plastic degenerates and leaks). No more than four gallons may be stored at home.

10 You must by law wear a crash helmet every time you use your motor bike.

11 Keep children away when you're doing something dangerous—in one third of DIY accidents it is the watching child who is hurt.

12 Never run an engine in a closed garage.

2 Don't

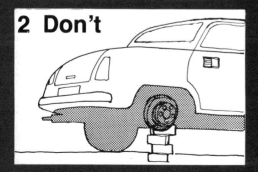

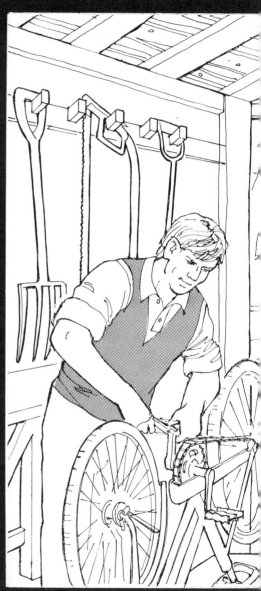

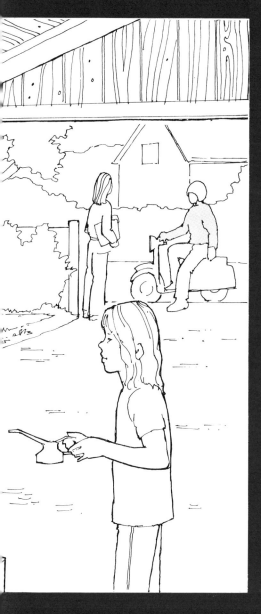

4 Don't

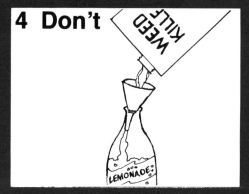

11 Don't

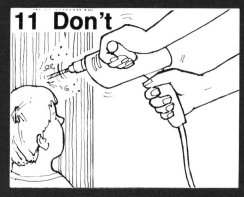

12 Don't

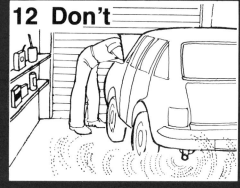

Gardens

1. Make sure ladders have a firm footing.

2. Don't be over-protective to older children.

3. Supervise small children all the time on swings.

4. Keep ponds fenced or covered if you have young children.

5. Make water butts safe.

6. Make sure paths and steps are even, especially for the elderly.

7. Teach children to recognise poisonous trees and shrubs.

8. Teach everybody to respect swimming pools.

9. Put out fires before going to bed.

10. Never throw inflammable liquids or aerosol cans on to fires.

11. Wear stout shoes or boots when mowing.

12. Clear lawn of stones and toys before mowing.

13. Never leave mowers unattended when the engine is running or when an electric mower is still plugged in.

14. When using power hedge clippers, keep flex over your shoulder out of your way.

15. Don't leave garden tools lying around—they're a danger to everyone.

16. Keep septic tanks properly covered.

17. Check deckchairs and garden furniture for safety after the winter.

18. Never adjust your mower or hedge trimmer while it is running.

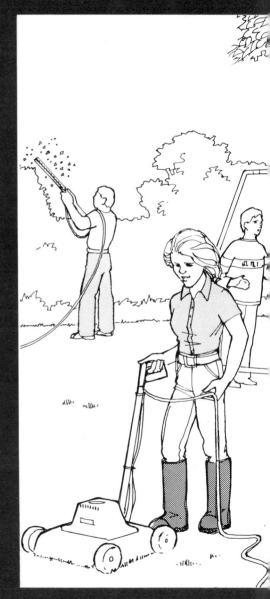

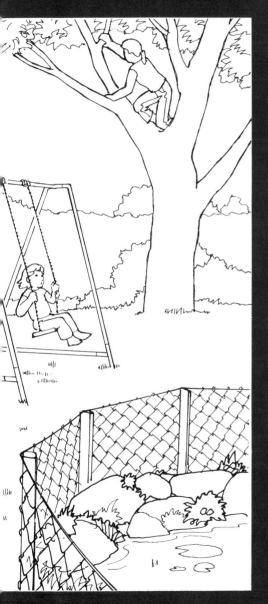

6 Don't

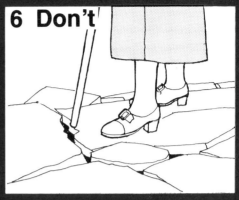

10 Don't

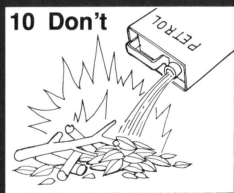

15 Don't

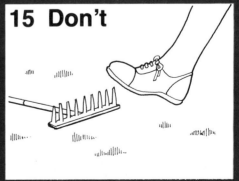

14 | Safety at home

Living room

1 Keep fires guarded. **Remember** it is illegal to leave a child under 12 in a room with an unguarded fire.

2 Keep pins, needles and scissors away from young children.

3 Make sure bookshelves can't be pulled over.

4 Put electric flexes where people won't trip over them but not under carpets.

5 Replace flexes immediately if they are at all chafed or worn.

6 Stand on something safe when dusting.

7 Unplug the TV when going to bed or leaving the house.

8 Never take the back off the TV or obstruct the ventilation slots.

9 Keep all plastic bags away from children. This includes the inner sleeves of records.

10 Never leave windows open without a safety catch where a young child plays.

11 Never put mirrors over the mantelpiece. Clothes could catch fire while looking in the mirror.

12 Don't leave small objects lying around with small children about—they may swallow them or put them in their ears or noses.

13 Beware of catching fingers under sash windows and in doors.

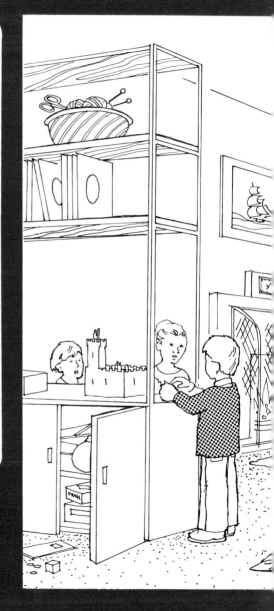

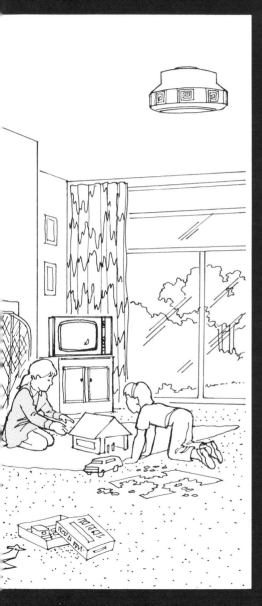

4 Don't

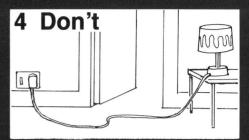

6 Don't

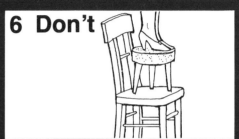

10 Don't

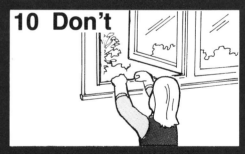

11 Don't

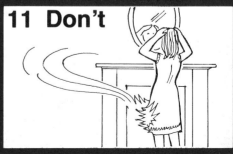

Bedrooms, hall, stairs and passages

1 Never move an oil heater when it is alight. Position it where it cannot be knocked over.

2 If you have young children, fit safety catches to all windows above ground level.

3 Electric convector heaters are safest for children's bedrooms.

4 When using paraffin heaters ensure that there is adequate ventilation.

5 Close medicine containers and return to medicine cupboard at once after use.

6 Don't smoke in bed.

7 Disconnect electric underblanket before going to bed.

8 Return electric underblanket to manufacturer for regular servicing. Never use for the very young or the old who wet the bed. They can, however, use electric overblankets.

9 Don't leave sleeping pills by the bed—repeated doses can be taken accidentally.

10 Loose mats should have non-slip backing strips.

11 Never carry too heavy or too big a load up or down stairs.

12 Use safety gates on the stairs with very young children about.

13 Good lighting is essential—no dark corners.

14 Don't store rubbish or anything inflammable under the stairs.

15 Never leave things lying on the stairs, and make sure stair carpet is well fixed and has no holes.

16 Keep a hand free to hold the rail or bannister.

17 Never meddle with gas or electrical installations. Call in an expert.

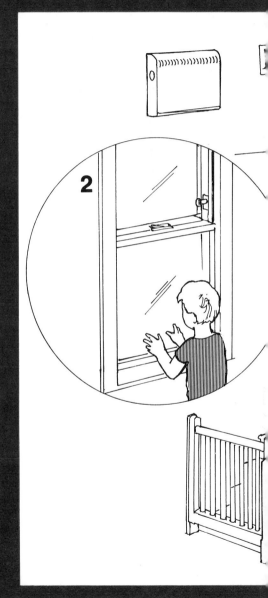

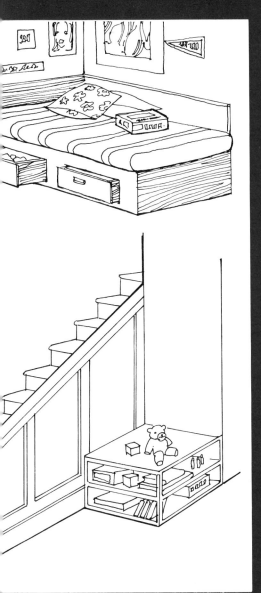

6 Don't

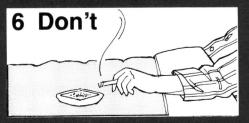

9 Don't

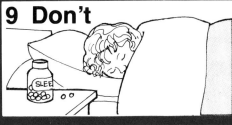

14 Don't

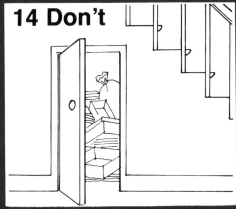

15 Don't

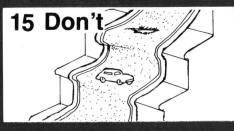

First aid or emergency care is exactly what it says it is. It is **not** medical treatment and you shouldn't compare what you can do with what a doctor would do. Nobody expects you to make **medical** decisions, simply common sense decisions that seem to be in the injured person's best interests at the time.
These are my top 10 rules for any emergency situation.

1 Look after yourself—don't do anything hazardous or thoughtless that puts you in danger or there could be twice the problem for someone else to cope with. Get the casualty and yourself away from hazards as soon as possible. Don't get trapped by collapsing buildings, gas, smoke or fire.

2 Look first for **essential** problems.
Check for: breathing
choking
bleeding
consciousness
Action on these can save life—anything else is a frill and can be done while awaiting professional help.

3 Get help as soon as the life-saving is under way. Don't try to do without professional aid—it's their job, they have the equipment and knowledge and are used to taking the responsibility when things go wrong. Tell the professionals over the phone how many casualties there are, what happened, exactly where you are, your telephone number and whether special equipment is needed.

4 Reassure the injured person and keep him as happy as possible under the circumstances. Combine confidence (which you may not feel) with kindliness.

5 Organise bystanders—don't let them stand around making remarks that could upset the casualty. 'Give him air' is a common cry that goes up in such situations. This is nonsense of course because the casualty will have plenty of air. What he does need is emotional 'air'—i.e. calm, reassuring care and not a crowd of fussing people standing around him.

6 If there are several casualties, decide quickly which most needs urgent attention and if necessary quickly show a bystander how to do artificial respiration or heart massage.

7 Don't worry yourself into doing **nothing** for fear of doing the wrong thing. You are, after all, not expected to know about all the conceivable complications that might arise from your actions. It's better to turn an unconscious person carefully into the recovery position and clear the airway every time, because 99 times out of 100 you'll be doing exactly the right thing. The other case in 100 will have a broken neck and you could possibly injure him further but this is the price we have to pay. Take the calculated risk—you'll wish someone would do so for you or for a member of your family.

8 Once you have carried out life-saving procedures, do nothing, unless you are absolutely sure of what you're doing. **Inactivity is the most difficult activity.** Harm can be done by piling blankets on injured people (which overheats them); giving drinks of tea to everyone in sight (dangerous as injured people vomit easily and may drown themselves in the tea you've just given); sitting people up (who should be kept flat because they may have a back injury); and taking people off into cosy front rooms 'in the warm' where they are overlooked by the emergency services or simply can't be found at all.

9 Take charge and organise. If you've read this book you'll be in a much better position to cope with problems than the average bystander, so protect the casualty from ill-informed actions. Ask others to help in other ways while you do the first aid. Of course, should there be a doctor or nurse in the crowd, they can take over.

10 Always stop when you see an accident unless professionals are already on the scene. The simple actions described in this book will enable you to save life and prevent further injury. Knowing what to do puts you in a privileged position but it also carries responsibilities. Don't pass by—one day it could be you or your family lying there.

How to tell

1 Put your cheek against the person's mouth and feel for breaths.
2 If breathing is not obvious, purse the person's lips and try cheek again.
3 Look for chest movements (may be difficult to see because of bulky clothes).

Breathing stopped

1 Lie the person on the ground.
2 See if there is anything in his mouth (vomit, false teeth, foreign body etc) that might be causing obvious obstruction. If so, remove it and lie him on his back.
3 Pull the chin upwards so that the person's head is bent backwards. With your left hand pulling the chin up, push the top of his head down with your right. This simple procedure opens the airway at the back of the throat and he may restart breathing. Once he does, put him in the **recovery position (a)** and stay with him, see pages 78–79.

If breathing doesn't restart at once

Start artificial respiration while someone else gets a doctor or an ambulance.

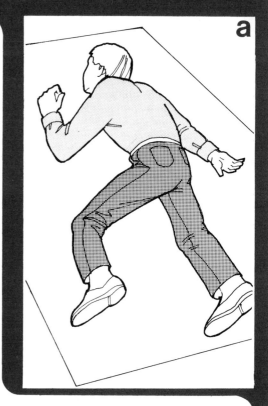

a

The best method by far is the **'kiss of life'** (mouth to mouth resuscitation)
1 Put the person on his back.
2 Tilt the head back as far as possible (nostrils then point directly upwards at you).
3 Cup one hand under his chin.
4 Put the heel of the other hand on his forehead so that the fingers of that hand can pinch his nose.
5b Use both hands together to lean the head back.

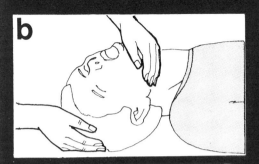

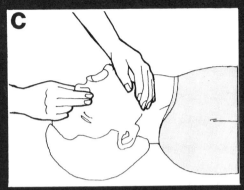

6c Pinch the nose shut.
7 Make sure the person's mouth is open.
8 Take a full breath yourself.
9d Apply your mouth to his, ensuring that there is a good seal all round.
10 Breathe into his mouth firmly and slowly—don't puff out hard. As you do this, the person's chest will rise.
11e Take your mouth away, breathe in fully and repeat the procedure.
12 While you are taking a breath in, the subject will breathe out spontaneously.
13 Repeat the breathing into his mouth and watch for spontaneous restarting of breathing as you turn your head away to breathe in yourself.
14 Try to 'blow' a breath into the victim about every 6 seconds. Be guided by common sense on this. For example, the first few breaths can be given much more quickly to try to get some oxygen into the person.
15 Stop when the person shows clear signs of starting to breathe but even then keep a close eye on his chest movements until professional help arrives.

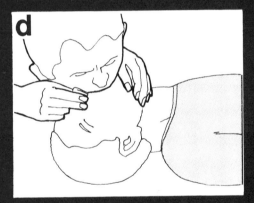

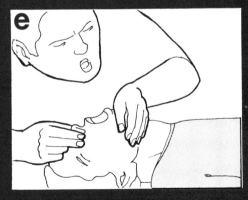

Some useful hints

1 Don't blow too hard (see page 21) as this may send air into the stomach and make the person vomit, which is dangerous for him and unpleasant for you.

2a Should he vomit, turn his head to one side and let the vomit dribble out of his mouth. Clean out the mouth and carry on with resuscitation.

3b If a child is the victim, seal your lips over both nose and mouth after positioning the head as before. **Only blow gently.** Be guided by what produces a rise and fall of the chest wall. In babies, use only the amount of air you can hold in your cheeks— **don't blow from your lungs.**

4 If the abdomen starts swelling up, you'll know you're blowing air down the gullet into the stomach instead of down the windpipe. Stop resuscitation for a moment, turn the child to one side, press firmly over the swollen stomach. This will probably force the air out.

5c Check that the person's heartbeat hasn't stopped by feeling in the neck for the carotid pulse from time to time.

How long to continue?

EITHER

until the person starts to breathe easily again. Never try breathing into someone who is already breathing spontaneously. It can be helpful though to give the odd helping breath if he is gasping or breathing irregularly

OR

until professional help arrives. This may take time, so get others to help you. Keep going until a doctor says the person is dead. Don't give up too readily, especially in cases of drowning or electric shock.

What about other methods?

The mouth to mouth method or 'kiss of life' is undoubtedly the most effective way of getting someone breathing again. One other technique is worth mentioning but the chances that you'll have to use it are slender and it should only be applied if the person has such severe facial injuries that you can't do mouth to mouth resuscitation.

The Sylvester method involves a kind of rhythmical pumping of the person's arms as he lies flat on his back. Start with his arms crossed over his upper abdomen and, kneeling down with your knees either side of his head, rock backwards and pull his arms upwards and outwards so as to expand his chest. Return his arms to the crossed position over his lower chest/upper abdomen. Repeat 12 times a minute.

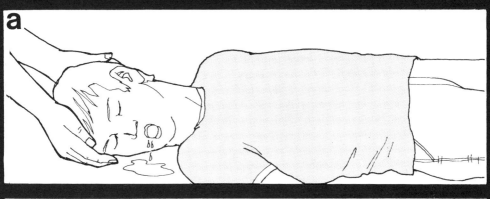

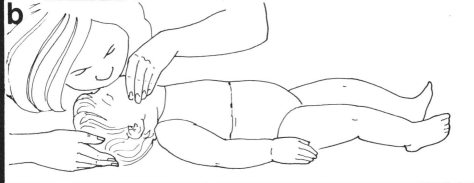

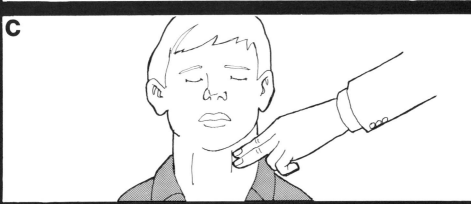

How to tell

1 Person unconscious.
2 Person looks pale or blue-grey.
3a The pupils of the eyes (the black part in the centre) are very large.
4b No pulse over the carotid artery (felt in the groove at the side of the Adam's apple).
5c No heartbeat heard on applying your ear to the left side of the breast bone.

What to do

1 Lie the person on his back on a hard surface. If on a bed, quickly but carefully lift him on to the floor.
2d Give one sharp, hard blow with the side of the hand over the lower left side of the breastbone. This may 'shock' the heart into re-starting spontaneously. Send someone else for an ambulance while you:
3 Start cardiac massage—BUT ONLY IF YOU ARE SURE THE HEART IS NOT BEATING.
4 Kneel on the person's right side facing him.
5e Put the heel of one hand over the lower half of the breastbone (not on its lower end). The rest of your hand shouldn't exert pressure on the chest at all.
6 Place the heel of the other hand on the back of the first hand.
7 Keep your arms straight and rock backwards and forwards. Don't apply pressure by bending your arms or you'll be exhausted within no time—let your body weight do the work. Keep your hands in position all the time.

In **adults**: Depress the chest wall about 5 cm (2 in), 60 times per minute.
In **children**: Use one hand only at 80 times per minute.
In **babies**: Use 2 fingers only at 100 times per minute and press higher up the breastbone so as not to damage the liver which is large and easily ruptured.

How long to continue?

1 Until the person looks a better colour.
2 Until his pupils reduce to normal size.
3 Until the neck pulse returns or he starts to recover.
If any of these signs is apparent, stop and check for the heartbeat or pulse.

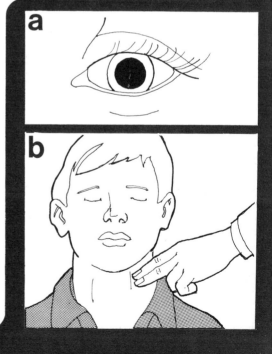

a

b

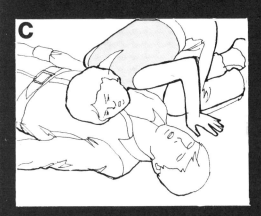

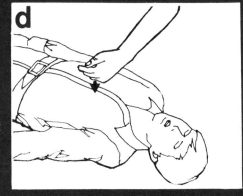

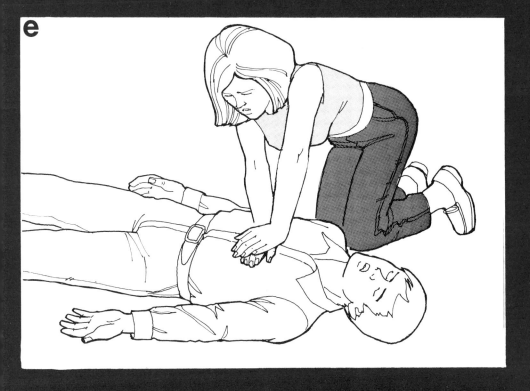

If you are alone:
1a Inflate the lungs quickly twice (as described on pages 20–21).
2b Do 15 heart compressions (as detailed above).
Repeat this circuit time after time while someone goes for help or an ambulance.

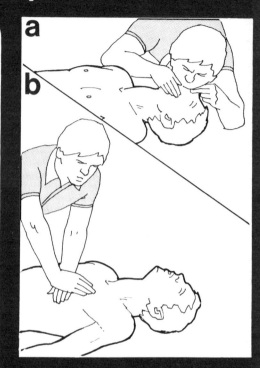

Don't go on compressing the chest of someone whose pulse has returned. Although breathing may stop on its own, the heart stopping also causes breathing to fail. So with someone whose heart has stopped you have a double problem.

When another person arrives:
One person should do mouth to mouth resuscitation (the kiss of life) while the other does cardiac massage (**c**).
Keep the sequence as follows:
You breathe 1 breath—he does 5 heart compressions—you do one breath—he does 5 heart compressions and so on until successful
OR until professional help arrives.
The person doing the breathing part should also check the neck pulse.

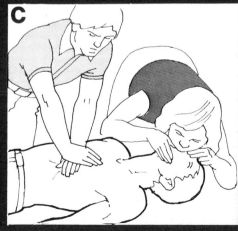

Why heart massage works

Contrary to popular belief, the heart lies almost centrally in the chest and not under the left nipple. If the breastbone is depressed sufficiently (about 5 cm (2 in) in an adult) the heart will be physically compressed between the breastbone in front and the spine behind. This is not the way the heart normally performs but is a useful first aid procedure. This is why when you do cardiac massage you must only press in the centre of the chest, over the breastbone. If you press over the ribs you may break them but worst of all you won't be doing anything useful to the heart so the whole thing will be a waste of time.

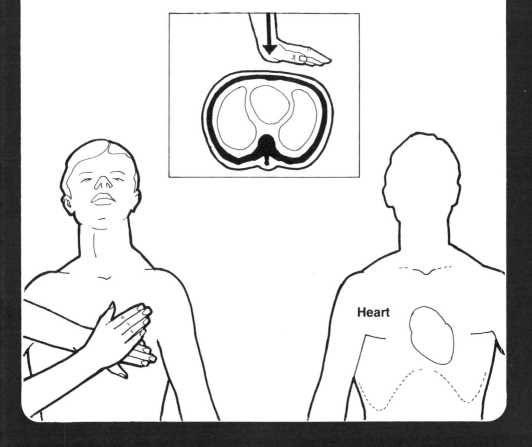

Heart

Some helpful thoughts:
1 For every stone of body weight we have approximately one pint of blood.
2a The average healthy adult can lose up to 850 ml (1½ pints) without serious effect. In children, half a pint can be critical.
3 When you cut yourself the amount of blood lost always looks a lot more than it actually is, so don't panic.
4b Severe bruising can remove more blood from the circulation than may a fair sized cut. For example, a fractured thigh can cause a loss of up to three pints of blood yet there is no visible bleeding.
5 Forget whatever you have been told about pressure points—they're hard to find in dressed people and even harder to keep pressure on for long periods.
6 Mild bleeding stops of its own accord because the body has a 'plugging up' mechanism that comes into play when the blood vessels are damaged. Simply apply firm pressure over the area until bleeding stops.
7 Stopping severe bleeding is essential, life-saving, and should be done as follows:
i Don't delay, do something at once. Get someone else to call an ambulance.
iic Raise the bleeding part where possible. This reduces the blood flow to some extent simply by reducing the effects of gravity. If you think the part might be fractured, don't raise it. (For how to tell, see page 36).
iiid Apply pressure to the wound. Use your fingers and thumb to close the edges of the wound together. Grab it hard—don't be afraid of hurting the person. **Don't waste time washing your hands.**

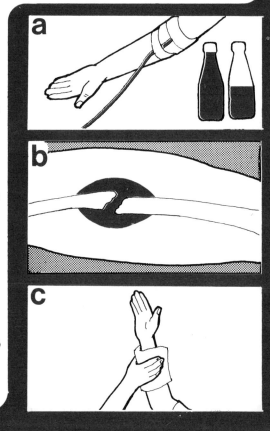

ive If this doesn't seem to be producing results, ask someone to get you a freshly laundered cloth of any kind, make it into a pad large enough to cover the wound and press it firmly on to the wound for 10 minutes. If you're on your own, use your handkerchief and tie it on as a dressing when you get tired of pressing it on. Don't worry too much about infection—bleeding is more dangerous at this stage.

vf If you have proper dressings handy, put on a sterile pad of gauze or wool and bandage the area firmly. Should blood seep through this dressing, apply more dressings on top and then more bandage. Don't undo it all or you'll dislodge any clots that are forming.

vi Never apply a tourniquet—this can cause serious damage in untrained hands and seldom works unless applied by an expert.

vii Rest the damaged part, elevated if possible.

viii Keep talking to the injured person and reassure him that all is well.

ix Keep a look out for the signs of shock. (See page 34 for action should this occur). **Signs to watch for are: pale, clammy skin; sweating; nausea; anxiety; rapid, shallow breaths; weak, thin pulse; faintness.**

x Hand over to professionals or take the person to hospital.

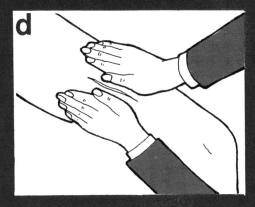

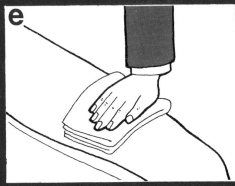

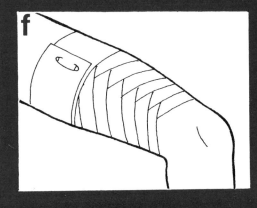

Could there be internal bleeding?

Any serious accident can be complicated by internal bleeding even though the injured person seems and feels well (at first anyway).

Invisible bleeding can be just as serious as visible bleeding.

Things to look for:

1 Bruising—especially over a large area or over the trunk
2 Dizziness
3 Cold, clammy, sweaty skin
4 Rapid, weak pulse
5 Difficult breathing
6 Frothy blood being coughed up
7 Severe abdominal pain
8 Evidence of a fracture (see page 36)

Action : Treat for shock (see page 34) and get professional help quickly. Dial 999.

Types of wounds
Graze:

A roughened area of skin which is bleeding or oozing fluid.

Clean around the area gently, dry and apply a dressing if it is likely to get dirty.

Simple incision:

Caused by sharp edge of glass, knife, razor etc. A very clean cut. If less than $1\frac{1}{2}$cm ($\frac{1}{2}$in) long, will probably heal well if you stop bleeding, pull edges together and apply adhesive dressing. Don't fiddle about with disinfectant. Wash your hands, clean the area around the wound, ensuring that none

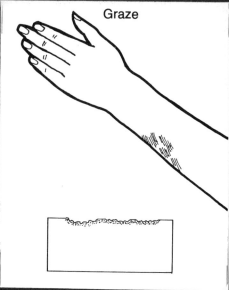

Graze

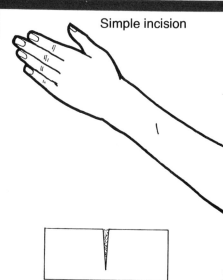

Simple incision

of the water gets into the open wound, dry it carefully, then apply the dressing. Other incisions need stitches. Stop bleeding by applying pressure. Apply a dressing and bandage if you have them. Go to hospital or call for an ambulance if the bleeding is severe.

Laceration:

A torn, rough and jagged wound.

These wounds are caused by rough spikes or other sharp things rather than by knife-like objects. They are much more difficult to treat and need hospital attention. Stop bleeding by applying pressure. Only remove large and loose pieces of glass or other debris—otherwise leave this to the experts. At hospital they will clean the wound, search for foreign bodies, carefully piece the edges together and stitch them. This sort of injury particularly calls for tetanus protection. Tell the doctor when you last had a tetanus injection. (See page 108)

Puncture:

A wound often with very little bleeding, caused by poking with a sharp tool, nail, needle etc. Such wounds seem trivial and yet need to be taken seriously because they can cause deep infection. See a doctor or go to hospital.

Bruise:

Caused by damage from a blunt object. If the area of bruising is very large, get medical help. If not, rest and local warmth are helpful.

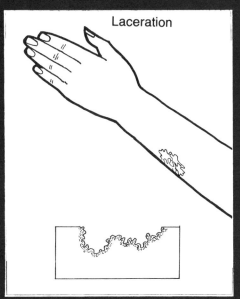

Laceration

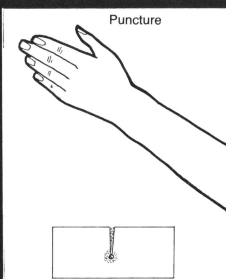

Puncture

Some special bleeding problems
Nose bleed (a):

1 Sit down, preferably at a table. Put a bowl under your nose on the table.
2 Grasp the soft part of your nose firmly between your thumb and index finger.
3 Lean your head forwards and hold your nose for 10 minutes—this cures the vast majority of nose bleeds.
4 Never ignore a nose bleed in someone who has hit his head or had a fall, especially if the nose is discharging clear fluid as well as blood. This is a sign of a fractured skull and needs immediate medical attention.
5 Once a nose bleed has stopped, don't blow or sniff. You'll dislodge the clot and have to start all over again.
6 If you have lots of nose bleeds, tell your doctor.

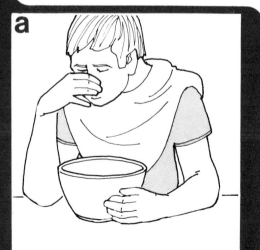

Bleeding from the back passage:

This is almost always caused by piles. See your doctor for advice. Never ignore bleeding from your back passage. If the bleeding is accompanied by a sharp pain, you may have torn the skin because you are constipated. Eat plenty of high fibre foods (vegetables, wholemeal bread, bran-containing breakfast cereals) and you won't be troubled again. This is also good treatment for early piles.

Bleeding tongue:

Sit as with a nose bleed. Grasp the tongue with a freshly laundered handkerchief. Press for 10 minutes.

Bleeding tooth socket:

Usually happens after a tooth extraction.
Don't wash out the mouth or you'll disturb clot formation. Sit up as for nose bleeding. Put a thick wad of gauze or similar material over the socket area and bite hard on it. Do this for 10 minutes and then gently remove the dressing. If bleeding persists, telephone the dentist who did the extraction.

Bleeding into the urine:

If your urine is bloody there is nothing you can or should do except tell your doctor. It can be caused by trivial or serious conditions but needs thorough investigation. (Beetroot, some sweets and some constipation medicines can make your urine red.)

Bleeding from the stomach:

Most likely caused by a bleeding ulcer. Blood in vomit can be red, brown or black like coffee grounds. The colour indicates how long it has been in the stomach. (It darkens with time.)
Keep the person lying down. Watch for shock (see page 34 for signs) and get medical help.
Beware of red foods when worrying about blood in vomit. It's usually easy to tell beetroot, red peppers and tomatoes from vomited fresh red blood if you look carefully.

Bleeding scalp:

The scalp is especially rich in blood vessels and bleeds profusely even from small cuts. Apply pressure to the cut area for 10 minutes using a freshly laundered handkerchief. If the bleeding doesn't stop (and it might well not, unlike other areas of the body) go to hospital for stitches. **Remember** that any wound of the scalp may be accompanied by a fracture of the skull. If you feel peculiar in any way, have difficulty with speaking or coordination, feel drowsy or have any watery or blood stained fluid from your nose or ears, get medical help at once.

Bleeding from the lungs:

The strain of repeated coughing can cause tiny streaks of blood to be coughed up. Heavier bleeding from disease or injury to the chest needs medical attention and is usually pink and frothy. If bleeding is heavy, go to hospital at once or call an ambulance.

Bleeding from the ear:

Any bleeding from inside the ear must be treated with respect. In any person who has fallen or possibly hit his head, think of a fractured skull if blood comes from the ear, especially if it is accompanied by clear, watery fluid. Get medical help.

Bleeding varicose veins (b):

Press over the bleeding point with or without a dressing. Raise the leg on a stool or chair as you lie on the floor. Remove stockings and garters and bandage a dressing or freshly laundered handkerchief over the area. Talk to your doctor about long term treatment of the varicose veins.

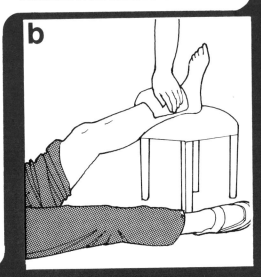
b

34 | Shock

What is it?

Emotional shock—feeling faint or weak, even to the point of fainting. Brought about by unpleasant sights, emotional trauma etc. This comes on quickly. **True shock**—a condition with many causes that affects body functions severely. It may end in death. For fainting see page 128.

What causes it?

1 Severe loss of blood—usually more than 850ml (1½ pints). Don't forget that a person can lose pints of blood internally (see Bleeding, page 30).

2 Loss of body fluid through the surface of burns or from prolonged diarrhoea and vomiting.

3 Severe bruising—even with no outward sign of blood loss there can be several pints of blood in the tissue around a fractured large bone.

4 Any condition that stops the heart beating (e.g. heart attack, electric shock).

5 Severe infection (for example a burst appendix).

6 Allergic shock.

Signs of a shocked person:

Pale or even grey
Cold to touch
Sweaty
Breathing in a rapid, shallow way
Pulse is fast and weak
Restless and anxious
Thirsty
Nauseated and may vomit
Unconscious

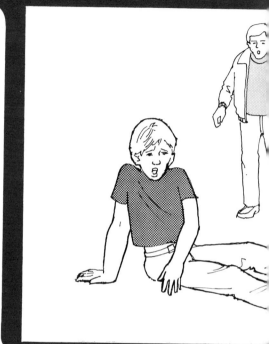

Action

If most of the above list are present, the victim is in a bad way and needs urgent medical help.

Get someone to call an ambulance.

Try to help the shock victim **before** he gets this bad.

For any severe injury, start preventing shock even before signs appear.

1 Stop bleeding. Press over the area and see page 28 for more details.

2 Remove him only from serious hazard—otherwise don't move him. If

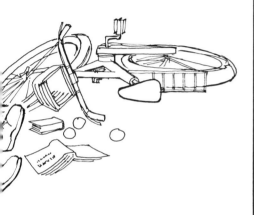

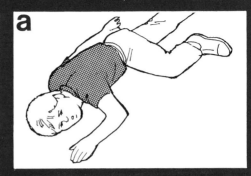

a

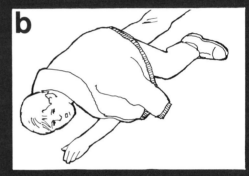

b

he's in the road—treat him there—and get others to keep traffic clear.

3a Place him in the recovery position (see page 79).

4 Cover up and dress any wounds to reduce distress.

5 Loosen tight clothing.

6b Keep him from getting chilled with a blanket or other light covering.

7 Do not apply heat or lots of blankets.

8 Reassure him; keep crowds away (give them things to do).

9 Never give anything by mouth to anyone in a severe state of shock (even if he is thirsty) or to anyone who is unconscious. Wet his lips with a damp cloth or your fingers dipped in water if he asks for a drink.

10 Never give alcohol or use hot water bottles—both draw blood (which is needed elsewhere for the vital functions of the body's organs) to the skin.

11 Watch breathing—resuscitate if it stops (page 20).

12 Feel pulse rate at neck. As shock develops, the pulse can double in rate (normal is around 70 beats per minute). If heartbeat stops, see page 24.

36 Fractures

What is a fracture?

A break in a bone. This can be caused by a direct blow or crushing injury or indirectly by transmission of force from one part of the body to another. For example, the collarbone can be broken by falling on an outstretched hand.

Types of fracture:

'Closed' or 'open'.

Closed fractures are of 3 types:

1a A greenstick fracture. Usually seen in children. In this type the bone is cracked on one side and buckled on the other. It heals quickly.

2b A simple closed fracture. Here the bone is broken, the ends may be displaced but the skin is intact.

3c A complicated fracture. A simple fracture but with complications involving nerves or blood vessels.

Open fractures (d) are more serious and look more 'obvious' because the bone actually pokes through the skin or has made a wound. These are more prone to infection.

How to tell if there's a fracture:

1e There is usually (but not always) pain over the fractured bone.

2f There may be swelling and/or bruising.

3g There is loss or severe restriction of use of the area affected.

4h Bone may poke through the skin.

5i There may be obvious deformity, bending, angularity, or floppiness of the affected part.

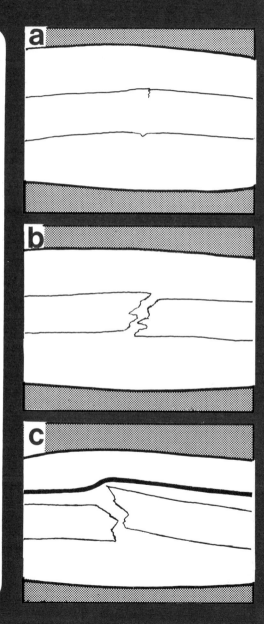

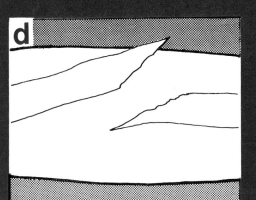

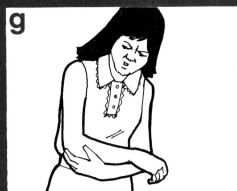

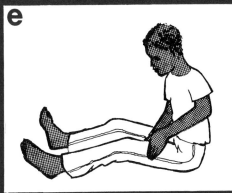

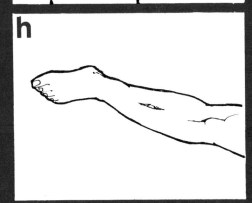

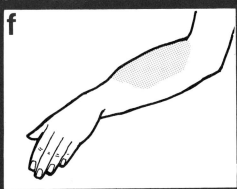

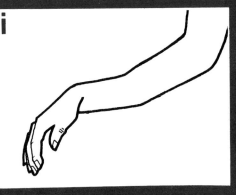

38 Fractures

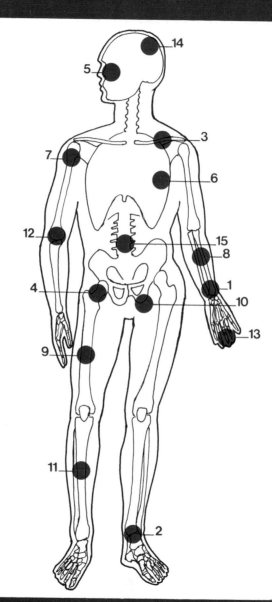

14
5
3
7
6
15
12
8
4
1
10
9
13
11
2

1 Wrist
2 Ankle
3 Collarbone
4 Hip
5 Nose
6 Rib
7 Upperarm
8 Forearm
9 Thigh
10 Pelvis
11 Shin
12 Elbow
13 Fingers
14 Skull
15 Back

General action

Ensure that the person is breathing (page 20), has a good pulse (page 24), isn't bleeding (page 32) and isn't going into shock (page 34).

Then make the person comfortable, tell him to keep still, cover open wounds and call an ambulance unless he seems well, has no obvious deformity and you can get him to hospital quickly in your own car. If moving him causes great pain, don't persevere but get an ambulance.

Give nothing by mouth to a person who may need an operation soon. **The commonest bones to be fractured are** (in approximate order of frequency depending on age):

1 Wrist	6 Rib	11 Shin
2 Ankle	7 Upperarm	12 Elbow
3 Collarbone	8 Forearm	13 Fingers
4 Hip	9 Thigh	14 Skull
5 Nose	10 Pelvis	15 Back

Action for specific fractures

General note: Most first aid books give great detail about splints, bindings and slings. These are mostly inappropriate for the ordinary man in the street to use. Moving people with fractures is a skill that has to be learned and practised. If in any doubt whatsoever, don't touch the person's damaged part unless he is in physical danger from life-threatening hazards such as gas, fire or collapsing buildings.

Never do anything to move or splint a compound (open) fracture, unless you have had training.

There are some simple things that are worth doing though, provided they don't cause the person undue pain. What is permissible varies from bone to bone so check first before doing anything. If you haven't any bandages then scarves, stockings or ties will do.

Upper arm, forearm, hand and wrist:
Signs:
Pain, swelling and tenderness over the affected area. If there is pain when the thumb and index fingers are pushed hard together (**a**), the small scaphoid bone in the wrist may be broken.
Action:
1 Put a pad of soft material between the chest and upper arm and gently pull the hand up to the level of the opposite nipple.
2 Safety pin the shirt or jacket sleeve to the lapel on the other side of the body.
3 Get the victim to support his bad arm's elbow with his other hand. Use a triangular sling if you have one.

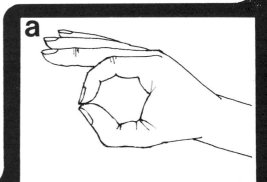

Collarbone:
Signs:
Pain etc over the collarbone. Run your finger along the line of the collarbone and feel for discontinuity of the curve. The person may be supporting his elbow to prevent a downward pull on the fracture. Mostly seen in children.

Action:
Use a triangular sling if you have one **OR** pin the sleeve as right **OR** simply get the child to support his own arm at the elbow.

Elbow:
Signs:
As for other fractures. Mostly seen in children. May be held bent or straight.

Action:
Keep the elbow in the position it is.
Don't bend a straight elbow to put it into a sling; don't straighten a bent one either or you may trap a blood vessel in the joint. If already bent, put into a sling (made from a triangular bandage if you have one) or pin the sleeve to the jacket. If straight, pin the arm to the side or immobilise it as shown.

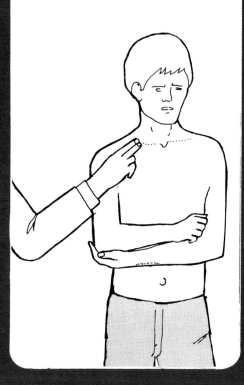

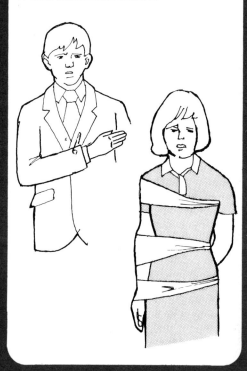

Ribs:
Signs
Pain over the ribs on breathing in or coughing. Shallow breathing because of pain.
Action:
Depends on severity. The person may be able to go to hospital in a car with minimal discomfort or may feel that a sling for the arm on the affected side helps (page 147). If the fracture is very severe, get medical help and do nothing to the chest. If a wound is present with fractured ribs, cover the wound to stop any noise of air sucking into the chest.

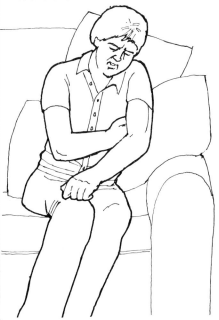

Hip:
Signs:
Pain in the hip or groin. The leg on the affected side looks shorter and the foot is turned outwards. Usually an old person.
Action:
Call an ambulance and follow the general action above.

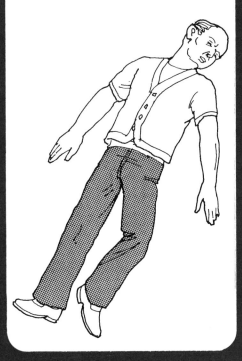

Thigh:
Signs:
Pain in the thigh. The leg looks shorter and the foot is turned outwards. There are often signs of shock because of blood loss into the tissues of the thigh. It is the strongest bone in the body so it is unlikely to be fractured except after a severe blow (except in the elderly in whom a relatively minor incident can cause a break).

Action:
Treat for shock. Don't move the victim. Get an ambulance.

Spine:
Signs:
Victims complain of pain in the back or neck and may have a loss of feeling, peculiar sensations or even paralysis of the legs (or arms and legs).

Action:
These people must be handled with extreme care. Never bend, twist or lift anyone with any of the above signs as you may paralyse him completely. Leave the person lying flat and check for breathing (page 20), bleeding (page 28) and shock (page 34). Tell the person to lie completely still and get an ambulance. Moving a person with a broken spine is a highly skilled business, so leave it to the experts.

Ankle and foot:
Signs:
Pain, deformity etc as in other fractures. Inability to put weight on that ankle and foot.

Action:
1 Take off the shoe and sock if you can do so extremely gently.
2 Gently elevate the leg on cushions or blankets to help reduce swelling. Get medical help.

Pelvis:
Signs:
The person is unable to stand, feels pain on moving his legs and is best lying down flat. He may feel like emptying his bladder. Usually occurs after a severe fall or crush injury.

Action:
Get expert help.

Jaw:
Signs:
Usually after a fall or crush injury. Serious because the same injury may have caused concussion, neck injury or brain damage.

Action:
1 Get an ambulance at once if he is unconscious.

2 If conscious: check breathing (page 20); bleeding (page 28) and prevent shock (page 34).

3a If all seems well, sit the person down at a table with a bowl underneath his chin on the table. Remove any broken teeth and dentures and get him to cup his chin in his hands.

4 Beware of the person becoming unconscious—never leave him alone.

5 If all is well, take him to hospital by car.

Skull:
Signs:
There is usually a scalp wound but not always. The person may be unconscious. Blood or pale watery fluid may come from the nose or ears. There may be bruising around the eye sockets or behind the ear.

Action:
1 As for unconsciousness (page 78) **even if the person is still conscious**.

2 Get expert help at once—call an ambulance. When getting the person into the recovery position ask someone to help you turn the head so as not to inflict further damage.

3b Look for other injuries—many head injury accidents also involve other parts of the body. If blood or watery fluid is coming from the ears or nose, position the head to let it run freely and apply a pad of absorbent material to soak it up. Stay with him until professional help arrives.

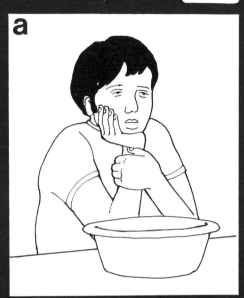

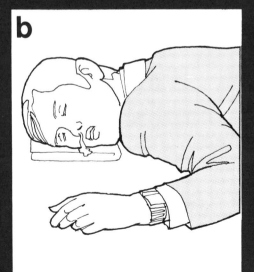

44 Sprains and dislocations

For muscle strains see page 100.

What is a sprain?

A condition in which ligaments around the joint are stretched or torn. Wrists and ankles are most commonly affected.

How do I know it isn't a fracture?

You don't. It's often very difficult even for doctors to tell. Sprains can be extremely painful so the degree of pain is nothing to go by. Often only an X-ray after careful medical examination will finally clear up the diagnosis.

If in doubt—treat as a fracture.

Action:

1 Rest the affected part.
2 Apply cold pads or ice in a polythene bag—these soothe the pain.
3 Support the joint with a crêpe bandage as follows:

Ankle:

1a Start with a crêpe bandage rolled up in one hand, support the ankle with the other and rest the foot on your knee.
2 Wrap one turn around the middle of the foot, working from the inside outwards.
3b Take the bandage across the top of the foot, around the back of the ankle and back underneath the foot, keeping up a good tension all the time.
4c Repeat the procedure in this figure of 8 fashion until the ankle is bandaged fully from the bottom of the toes to just above the ankle.
5 Secure the bandage and elevate the foot on pillows or blankets.

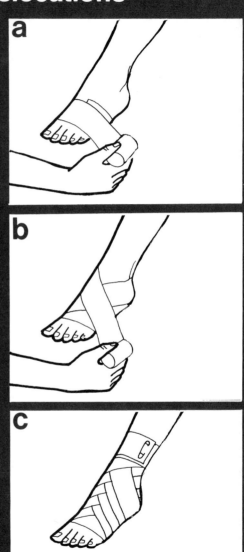

Knee:

1d Start below the knee and put one turn of the crêpe bandage around the leg just below the knee cap from within outwards.

2e Do a figure 8 with one turn alternately above and below the knee until the whole area is covered.

3f Overlap the bandage $\frac{1}{2}-\frac{2}{3}$ of its width at each turn and secure with a piece of tape, a safety pin or a bandage clip.

NOTE. When applying any elastic supporting bandage, ensure that it goes on firmly enough to give support but not so tightly that it impairs blood flow. If the part distant to the bandaged joint goes pale, blue, tingles or gives the person any other sensations, remove the bandage and apply it less tightly.

What is a dislocation?

A more serious sprain which has not only torn the ligaments but has displaced the bones of the joint. The commonest joints involved in dislocations are the fingers, jaw, shoulder and elbow.

Diagnosis may be difficult without X-rays but the joint may look deformed.

Action:

1 Treat as if it were a fracture (there may indeed be a fracture too).

2 Never try to replace dislocated joints.

3 Make the person comfortable and get medical help. If there is any numbness, tingling or other strange sensation in the affected limb, get the person to hospital as quickly as possible.

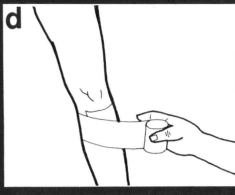

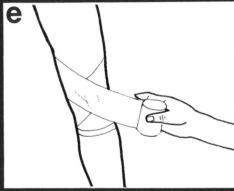

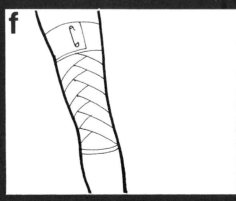

46 Heart attack

What is it?

Sudden damage to the heart's muscle which renders it less able to carry out its function as a pump. Some heart attacks are so severe that they stop the heart altogether; others render the person severely ill for a time but allow him to recover later; and others are so minor that they may cause only slight discomfort in the chest.

Signs:

1a Severe sudden pain in the chest. Usually the pain is central and described as 'crushing', 'gripping', or 'a tightness'. It is rarely sharp or knife-like.

2b Pain down the arms or into the neck.

3c The person looks pale, sweaty, anxious and has a rapid and perhaps irregular pulse.

4d Breathlessness.

5 If the heart attack is very severe, there may be no pulse or heartbeat.

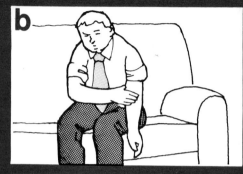

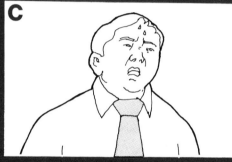

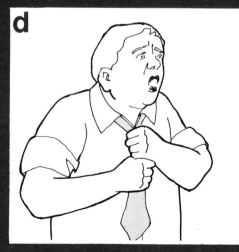

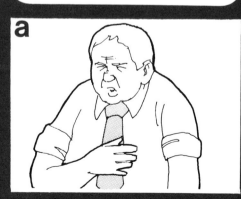

ANY PERSON COMPLAINING OF ANY OF THESE THINGS, EVEN IN ISOLATION, (EXCEPT FOR BREATHLESSNESS) NEEDS URGENT MEDICAL HELP.

Action.

Is the person conscious and cooperative?

If **yes**:

1e Sit him up at an angle of 45° in a bed or armchair or against a wall if out of doors.

2 Send for a doctor or ambulance, or get someone else to.

3 Get him to take a tablet of trinitrin if he carries them around with him for angina.

4 Loosen his clothing so that he can breathe easily.

5f Dry his face of sweat.

6 DON'T FUSS AROUND—KEEP PEOPLE AWAY.

7 Sit and talk reassuringly to him until professional help arrives.

If **no**:

1 Lie him down flat.

2 Loosen his collar and other restrictive clothing.

3g Feel for a pulse in the neck or place your ear on the left side of the breastbone and listen for the heartbeat. If none is heard, start resuscitation, see page 24). If the heartbeat is present, keep a close watch while someone else goes off for help. Stay at hand in case the heart or breathing stops. If breathing stops, proceed as on page 20.

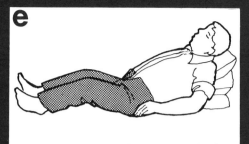

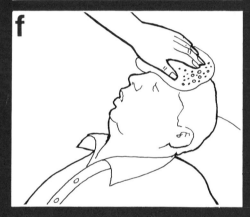

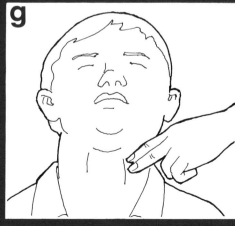

After a heart attack:

1 Always take your medicines as prescribed—no more and no less.
2 Keep your weight to a level that is right for your height. If in any doubt, ask your doctor.
3 Never overeat—an overfull stomach can cause pressure on the heart.
4 Don't rush around after meals.
5 Cut down, or preferably stop smoking altogether.
6a Take regular, controlled exercise but stop if you get chest or arm pain. Some people take up jogging after a heart attack with beneficial results.
7 Don't think of yourself as a cardiac cripple—millions of men in the West are leading happy and fruitful lives after a heart attack.
8 Don't give up sex. Studies show that the vast majority of heart attack patients can indulge in sexual activity without any fear of overstraining their hearts . . . BUT wait for 8 weeks after your heart attack before you start!
9 Get good restful sleep.

Prevention

Heart attacks kill an increasing number of people every year. One in three middle aged men today dies of a heart attack and the victims are getting younger and younger. Certain factors seem to increase the risk: 1) cigarette smoking; 2) high blood pressure; 3) high blood cholesterol (open to debate); 4) obesity; 5) lack of exercise; and 6) stress.

What to do

1b Stop smoking. If you smoke 20 or more cigarettes a day, you double your chance of having a heart attack.
2c Have your blood pressure checked by your doctor and keep to his treatment if it is high.
3d Cut down on fatty meat; use soft margarine instead of butter; use corn or sunflower oil for cooking; avoid cream; eat fewer than 3 eggs per week; cut down on pastries, cakes and biscuits; eat more fruit and vegetables; and eat wholemeal bread and wholemeal flour products. The advice here on cutting down on cholesterol-rich foods is currently under scrutiny but it will do no harm to reduce cholesterol-containing foods. Do not cut them out altogether though.
4e Get your weight down to what your doctor suggests. Start by cutting your sugar intake by half and eventually

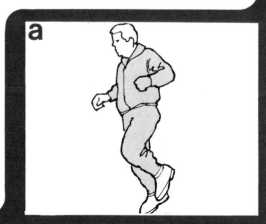

a

cutting it out altogether. This alone will reduce your weight surprisingly quickly.

5 Sedentary people have 3 times the chance of having a heart attack than active ones, so take regular exercise. Active people have 3 times the chance of surviving their first heart attack compared with inactive ones. Walk or jog regularly (2–3 times per week) in such a way as to raise your pulse to 120 beats per minute or more. Anything less than this cannot be considered to be 'protective' exercise. Having said this, take care not to exercise too much too soon, but work it up gradually.

6 Stress, especially in the presence of other risk factors, can be an important trigger. Avoiding stress can be difficult but it's worth trying to steer clear of the things that upset you or cause tension at work.

REMEMBER A heart attack doesn't just happen to other people—it could happen to you.

c

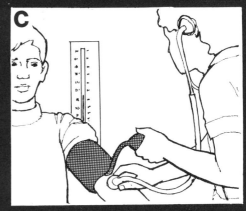

d

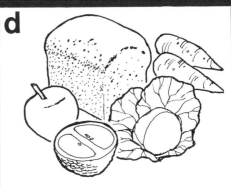

b Don't

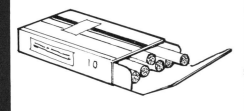

e

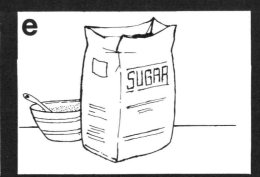

Adults usually choke on food, children also on foreign bodies such as coins, buttons and boiled sweets.

How to tell:
Children—
The child chokes, coughs and possibly goes blue.

Action
1a A very small baby can be held upside down and smacked on the back.
2b For an older child, lie him over your knee or over a chair and slap him hard on the back with the flat of the hand between the shoulder blades. This should dislodge the object and make him cough it up. If this doesn't work at once, try the Heimlich method:
ic Get behind the child and place your arms around his waist.
iid Clench one of your hands into a fist over the child's stomach between the navel and the rib cage.
iii Grip the clenched fist with the other hand.
iv Press your hands strongly against the abdominal wall, pressing slightly upwards. This sharp pressure drives the air out of the lungs suddenly and carries the obstructing object up through the windpipe.

Adults—
If you choke yourself it's very difficult to explain what's wrong simply because you can't speak. **Point to your throat repeatedly—(e)—someone will soon get the message** (see below). Should an adult choke on something, decide if he is simply coughing and spluttering. If so
1 Slap him on the back if he wants help but otherwise leave his cough reflexes to cope—they usually do.
2 Get him to try to breathe slowly and deeply. This reduces spasm of the windpipe and will release the choking object.

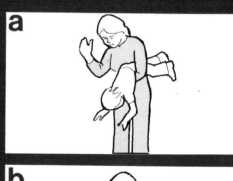

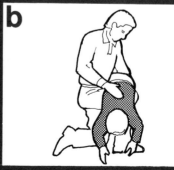

If the person is so obstructed that he's going blue.

1 Open his mouth to see if you can hook out the obstruction with your finger. It is usually too far back for this but it's worth looking quickly.

2 Get him on the floor and turn him on his side.

3f Slap him firmly on the back between the shoulder blades. This will almost always dislodge the foreign body.

If this doesn't work, use the Heimlich method (see below).

Fishbone in throat. If the person is choking really seriously, treat as adult choking. If not:

Do not try to reach into the throat to pick the bone out.

Do not give cotton wool sandwiches or other bulky remedies to swallow. Neither of these procedures works.

It's often difficult to know if you have in fact swallowed a bone or not as fishbones often simply scratch the lining of the throat yet give an impression of being stuck there. If all is well after an hour or two, the chances are it was simply a scratch. If things seem to be getting worse, go to hospital so that a doctor can look down your throat.

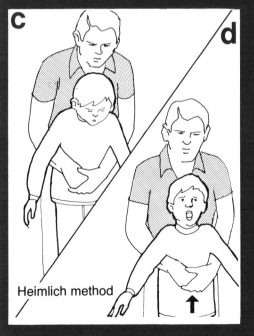

Heimlich method

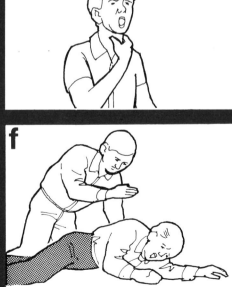

Why electricity is dangerous:

1 Electricity makes muscles contract as it enters the body (as when touching a live wire) or when breaking contact with the body (as when switching off the source of electricity). As it passes through the body tissues it can harm them but most important at home, it makes the muscles contract at 50 cycles per second—the frequency of alternating current in domestic appliances.

This means that if you grasp a faulty electrical appliance, your hand muscles may go into contraction around the handle and you'll be unable to let go of the thing that is giving you the shock.

2 Wet skin is especially efficient as a conductor, so never handle electrical appliances with wet hands and never have electric fires in bathrooms or kitchens within range of water.

3 As electricity passes through the body it damages tissues, causes clotting in blood vessels, injures brain and nervous tissues and can paralyse breathing and heart muscles. This is why it is so dangerous.

4 Electricity can kill instantly or can knock the person unconscious.

What to do:

Stop the contact with the electric current. You can do this by:

1a Switching off the supply at the wall socket.

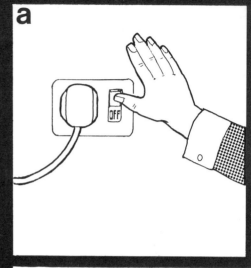

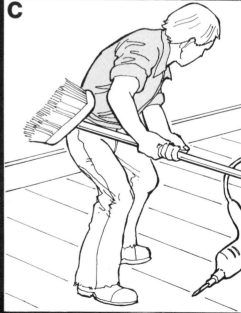

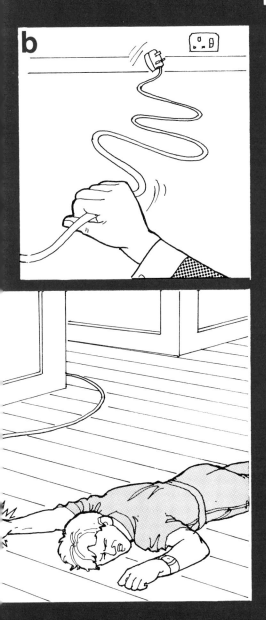

2b Pulling the cord hard so that the plug flies out of the socket.

3c Knocking the patient away from the source with an insulating object such as a wooden chair or a broomstick. This is often difficult to do. Whatever you do, DON'T TOUCH THE PERSON YOURSELF UNTIL HE'S CLEAR.

Once clear:

1 Do artificial respiration if breathing has stopped (see page 20).

2 Do heart massage if there is no heartbeat (see page 24).

3 Call an ambulance at once for anyone who has received a shock bad enough to make him lose consciousness. Some people seem well after an electric shock and then go downhill quickly, so don't be lulled into a false sense of security.

4 If many people are involved, attend to those whose breathing or heartbeat are affected first.

5 Perform resuscitation procedures for longer than normal because sometimes an electrocuted person revives after a surprisingly long time.

High voltage shocks

There is nothing a member of the public can do in cases of shock from high-tension leads, overhead cables, train conductor rails or high voltage power lines.

1 Keep people well away as this high voltage electricity jumps gaps and will 'find' any metal you're wearing.

2 Alert the authorities. Dial 999.

Lightning
To avoid being struck by lightning:

1 Keep away from trees, towers, small buildings, wire fences or any other projecting objects and don't ride a bicycle or other metal machine.
2 Shelter in a dense wood, under a cliff face or in a hollow in the ground. If you are sheltering under an isolated tree in a thunderstorm, keep well away from the trunk. You're safest of all in a car with a metal roof or in a building with a lightning conductor.

Help for those struck by lightning

As for electric shock. (See page 53, but of course you can't switch the current off). All efforts at revival should be prolonged as temporary nerve paralysis may delay recovery.
NOTE. There is no electricity left in the body after a lighting strike.

Prevention:

1 Never tamper with electrical appliances unless you are an expert.
2 Have electrical appliances serviced regularly.
If in doubt about the safety of any appliance or if you have any electrical emergency, phone your local 24 hour electricity service. Look under Electricity in the phone book.

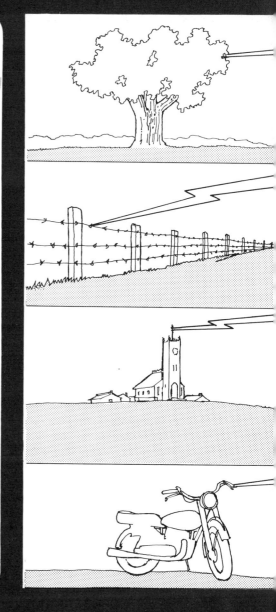

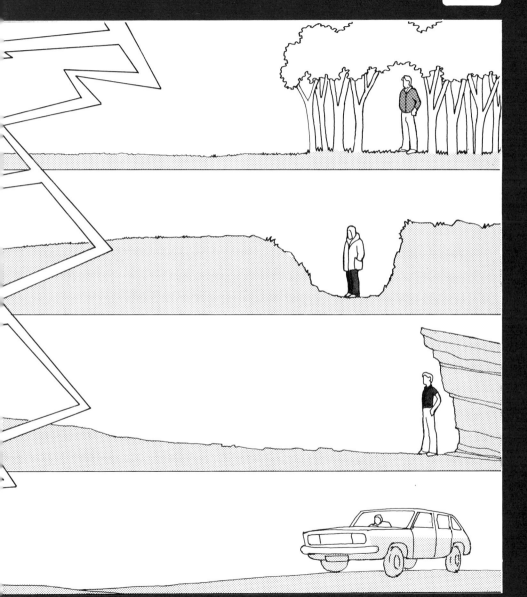

See page 72 for Fire.

General action:

1 Remove the source of burning or scalding.
2 Cool the affected area at once.
3 Treat shock if present (see page 34)
4 Get medical help if the person is severely ill.

Don't

1 Put cotton wool or any other fluffy dressings on to the burn (as they stick and are very difficult to remove).
2 Put grease, oily creams or butter on the wound. Leave blisters alone (if you burst them, you're encouraging infection).

What to do:

1a Place the part under running cold water for several minutes, or until the pain is relieved.
2 Gently remove rings, bracelets and other constricting things if possible from the affected area before swelling makes this difficult or impossible.
3b If you can't put the burnt area under water, drench it with water from a container and apply soaking towels.
4 Don't use iced water—this can be painful in itself.
5 Don't spray with a shower either. This can be extremely painful and may further damage the tissues.
6c Don't pull off any clothing around the burnt area unless the burn has affected only a small, confined area. Never pull away adherent charred clothes from flesh—this is an expert job.

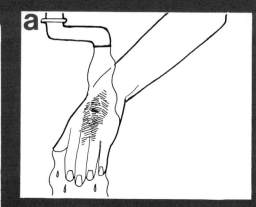

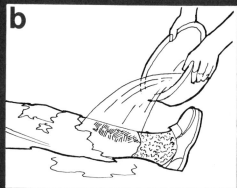

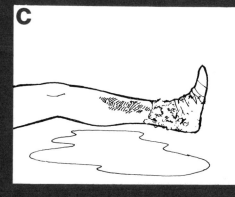

7 Once the area has been cooled, you can gently remove clothing from the affected area around the scald. This goes for chemical burns too. Be careful not to burn yourself with chemical-soaked clothes.
8 Decide whether the person needs medical attention.

Is medical attention needed?:
No, if:
the scald or burn is small (less than 2.5cm (1in) across), shallow, easily covered by a dressing and the person is well.
Yes, if:
1 the victim is a child;
2 the burn is large and especially if it involves areas of the body that move (around joints for example); affects the face; affects the palm or fingers or cannot easily be covered by a dressing;
3 the person is in shock or **if you are at all worried**;
4 caused by a chemical, electricity or molten metal (eg solder).
Be prepared to treat shock and to call an ambulance if the victim has 10% or more of his body burned or scalded.

For burns that you can treat:
1 Dry the area carefully.
2 Apply a dry dressing (not of cotton wool), preferably a non-adhesive burns dressing from your first aid box.
3 Bandage the area lightly to hold the dressing in place.
4 Keep the burnt part elevated to reduce swelling.

5 Give the person a painkilling drug in the full recommended dose if the pain is bad.
6 If the burn gets infected (red, pussy, weeping or increasingly painful), **get medical help**. Infection will produce scarring later.

For burns you cannot treat:
1 Lie the victim down and make him comfortable.
2 Give only tiny sips of water—any more may cause vomiting.
3 Keep calm and reassure him.

Some useful hints:
1 Remove clothes drenched in boiling fat, water or steam as soon as possible.
2 Remove clothes drenched in chemicals. If necessary cut them to get them off quickly. Wash the area with plenty of running water.
3 Take any electrical burn to a doctor.
4 Treat severe friction burns as other burns.
5 Scalds in the mouth can be helped by sucking ice.
6 If chemicals enter the eye, wash it out with water **at once**. Get the person to hold his face under water and blink or put the eye under **gently** running water. Protect the uninjured eye. Go to hospital quickly.
7 Sunburn victims need cool, shade, fluids to drink (small sips) and soothing cream (or calamine lotion). Get medical help for severe cases (see page 139).

58 Poisoning

What is a poison?

Anything which when taken into the body affects it adversely. Poisons can be tablets taken in excess (of which the commonest are painkillers, sleeping tablets and iron tablets); fruits and plants (eg mushrooms and berries); chemicals (eg weedkillers, domestic cleaning fluids and turpentine substitute (turps); bites (such as those from a snake); gases (like coal gas or industrial gases that are absorbed through the lungs); and agricultural pesticides that are absorbed through the skin.

It's usually obvious what sort of poisoning is involved, so we'll look at them group by group.

Swallowed poisons

Usually a child. It's difficult to know how much was swallowed unless you know how full the container was in the first place.

1 Any swallowed poison must be treated seriously. Get medical help as soon as possible. Ask someone to telephone for an ambulance or take the person to hospital by car at once.

2a Always take the container along with you so that the doctor can identify the poison and so possibly remedy it quicker. Tell the ambulance people what has happened and ask their advice.

3 Don't delay because children can go downhill very quickly even though they seem all right at first.

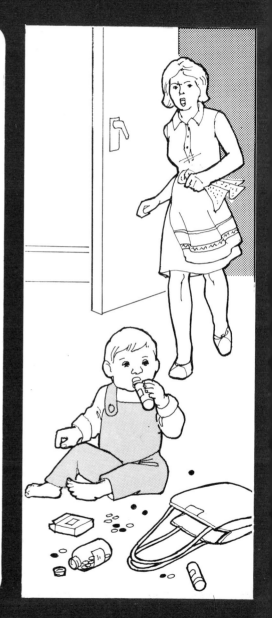

While awaiting medical help:

1 Remove excess poison from the mouth, keeping pills, berries or containers for the doctor to see.

2 If the person is conscious, ask what he took. Do this quickly in case he lapses into unconsciousness rapidly.

3 If the person is unconscious, turn him into the recovery position (see page 78) so that he won't suffocate or vomit. Keep any vomit to show the doctor.

4 Because many poisons adversely affect breathing, keep a close watch on the person. Should he stop breathing, give artificial respiration as on page 20.

5 If the person is conscious and has swallowed a corrosive substance, get him to drink water or milk to preserve the lining of the mouth (which can also be washed out) and to dilute the stomach contents. Remove any soaked clothing. You'll know if the poison is corrosive by the chemical burning and white discolouration it leaves on the mouth, lips and clothes.

6 Never give anything by mouth to an unconscious person no matter what you think he's taken.

7 Never make a person vomit if he has taken anything containing petrol, turpentine substitute or anything corrosive such as strong acids and alkalies. The substance will already have done plenty of damage going down and can only do more on its way up. Give these people milk or water to drink as this helps protect the stomach lining and to some extent prevents absorption of the chemical.

8 Never give salt water to make the person vomit. If the person has taken poisons other than corrosives, thrust three fingers well down the back of his throat to make him vomit. Little children can be held upside down as this is done. The person may even be able to make himself sick like this.

9 Never try to make anyone vomit if he is unconscious.

10 Keep a close watch on the person until help arrives.

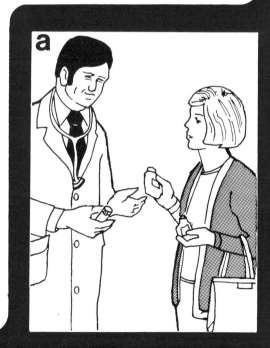

Some commonly swallowed poisons:

All of these should be kept away from children. Although they rarely kill, they can cause many unpleasant effects and worry both child and parent.

After shave lotion
Alcohol
Ammonia
Animal medicines
Antifreeze
Bleach
Brake fluid
Carpet cleaning fluids
Caustic soda
Detergents
(including bubble bath and washing-up liquid)
Disinfectants
Dyes
Fertilizers
Fire lighters
Garden chemicals
Glues
Insecticides
Lavatory cleaners
Lighter fuel
Medicines
Metal polishes
Methylated spirit
Mothballs
Nail varnish and
Paint and paint
strippers
remover
Paraffin
Perfumes
Petrol
Rat poisons
Shampoos
Turpentine substitute
(turps)
Weedkillers

Drugs are among the commonest causes of accidental poisoning in children. Aspirin, other painkillers, iron tablets, anti-depressants and sleeping pills are drugs which if taken in excess lead to serious illness or even death in children. Always keep medicines locked away out of the reach of children, preferably in a proper medicine cabinet. Many medicines come in foil strips with each tablet sealed safely away from children. If you have loose tablets, buy child-resistant containers with screw tops that can be undone by adults but not by children. Chemists sell bottles like this—ask at your local shop.

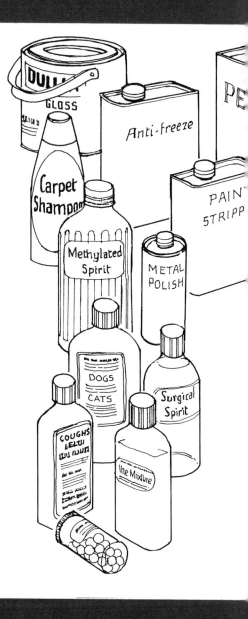

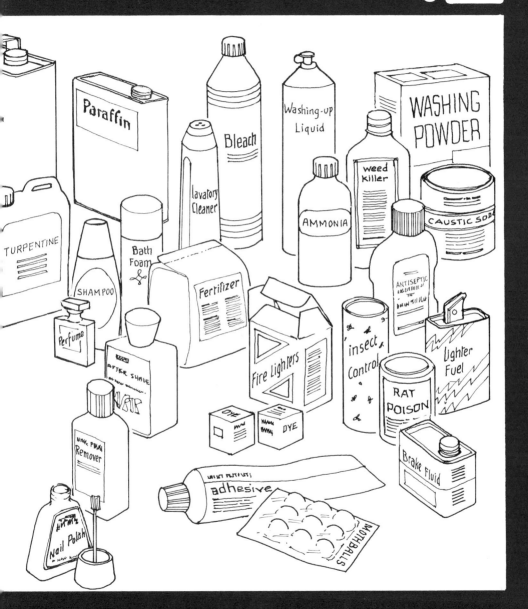

Some poisonous plants:

There are surprisingly large numbers of poisonous plants in the UK. The best rule is to teach your children never to suck or eat anything unless given to them by their parents or by other adults whom they know. Most of the poisonous plants listed below are unpleasant to eat and so are difficult to consume in large enough quantities to be harmful but even so—play safe with children.

Older children can be taught which plants are dangerous but even they should be taught not to eat anything.

Should your child swallow anything but the smallest amount of any of these plants, get medical help but don't panic. In the last 13 years there hasn't been a death from poisonous plants reported to the National Poisons Information Service in Britain.

Some common examples:

Poisonous garden plants:

Aconite (all of the plant)
Broom (seeds and pods)
Bryony (berries)
Cotoneaster (berries)
Daffodil and narcissus bulbs
Daphne (berries)
Deadly nightshade (berries)
Hemlock (young leaves and unripe fruit)
Honeysuckle (berries)
Laburnum (seeds and pods)
Laurel (leaves and berries)
Lupin (seeds and pods)
Potato (fruits and green tubers)
Pyracantha (berries)
Rhubarb (leaves)
Yew (berries)

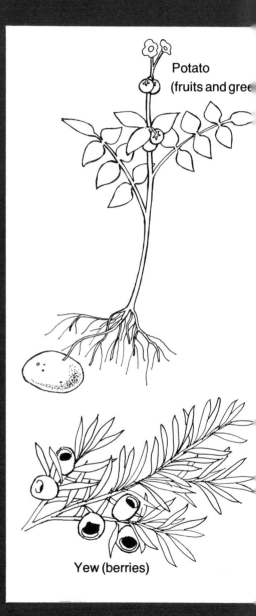

Potato
(fruits and gree

Yew (berries)

s)

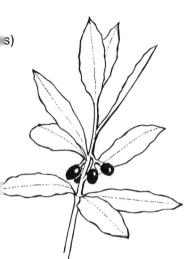

Laurel (leaves and berries)

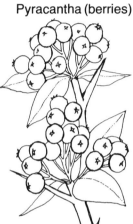

Pyracantha (berries)

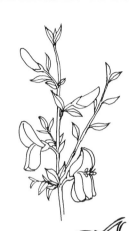

Broom (seeds and pods)

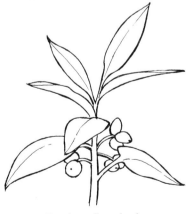

Daphne (berries)

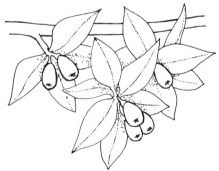

Cotoneaster (berries)

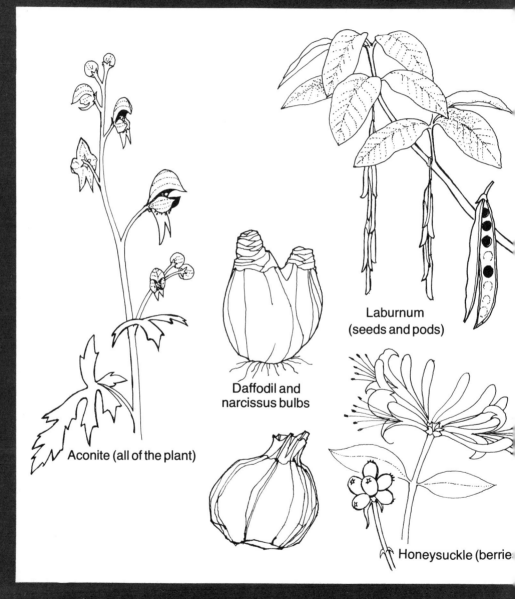

Aconite (all of the plant)

Daffodil and narcissus bulbs

Laburnum (seeds and pods)

Honeysuckle (berrie

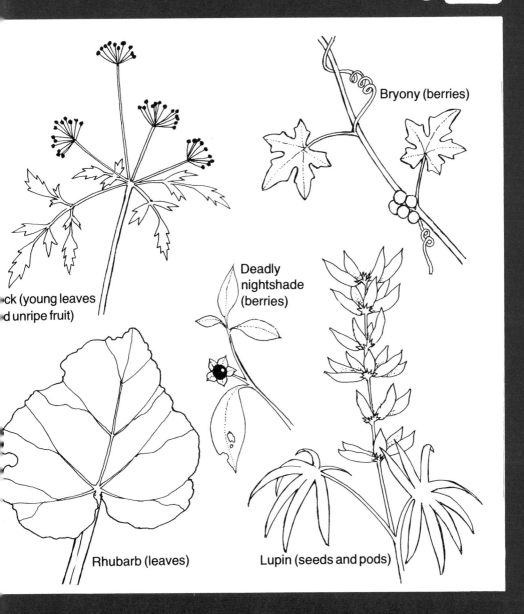

Bryony (berries)

...ck (young leaves
...d unripe fruit)

Deadly
nightshade
(berries)

Rhubarb (leaves)

Lupin (seeds and pods)

Poisonous countryside plants

Arum lily (berries and whole plant)
Deadly nightshade (berries)
Foxglove (whole plant)
Fungi (mushrooms and toadstools) — especially
  Death cap
  Destroying angel
  Fly agaric
  Fools' mushroom
  Panther cap
  Red-staining inocybe
Ivy (berries)
Mountain ash (rowan) (berries)

Mountain ash (rowan) (berries)

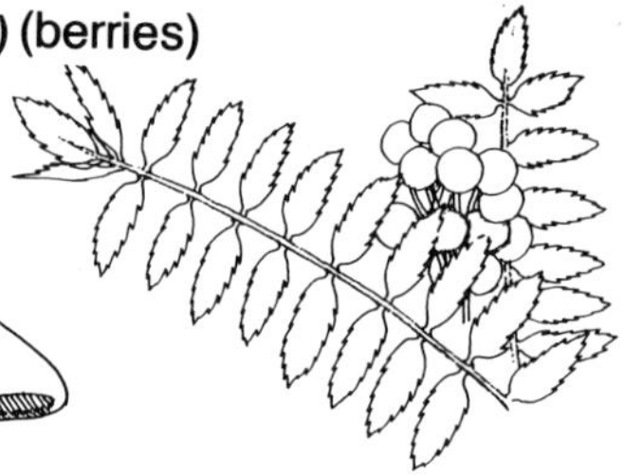

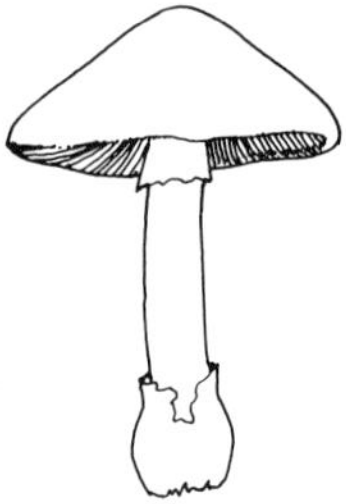

Fool's mushroom

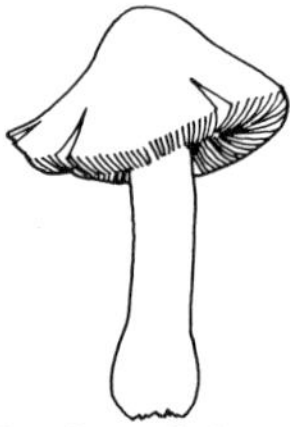

Red-staining inocybe

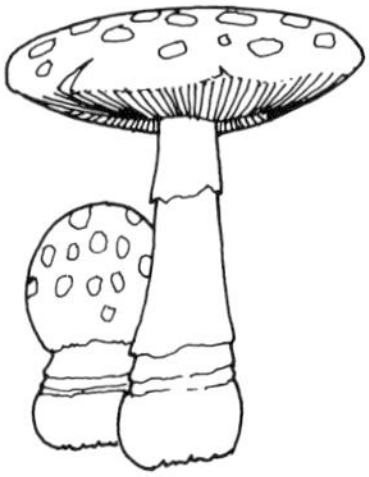

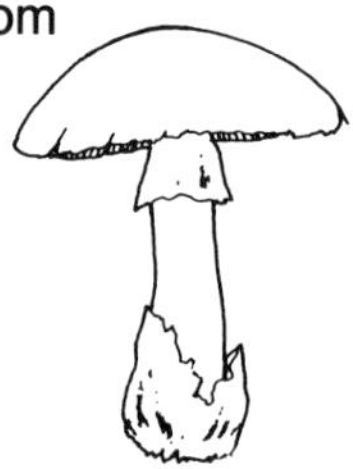

Fly agaric

Death cap

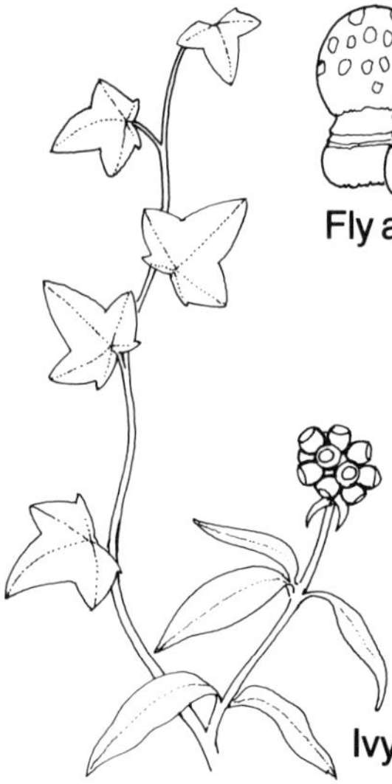

Ivy (berries)

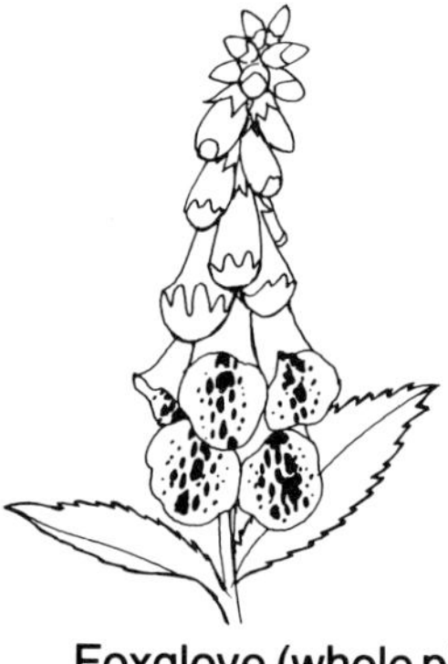

Foxglove (whole plant)

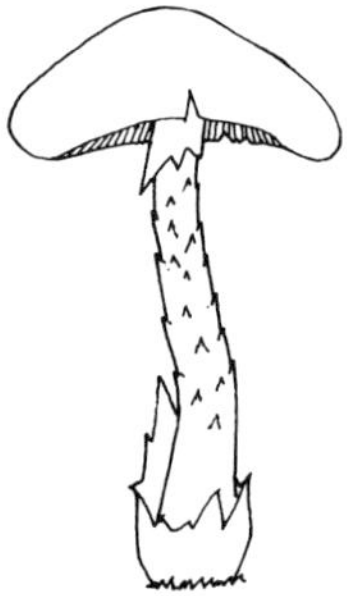

Destroying angel

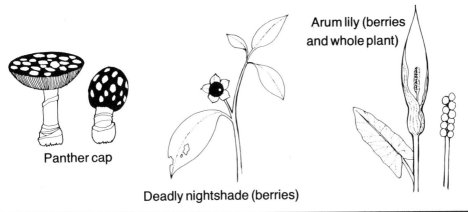

Arum lily (berries and whole plant)

Panther cap

Deadly nightshade (berries)

Poisonous indoor plants:
Dumb cane (sap)
Oleander (whole plant)
Poinsettia (dangerous sap)
Solanum or 'Christmas cherry' (berries)

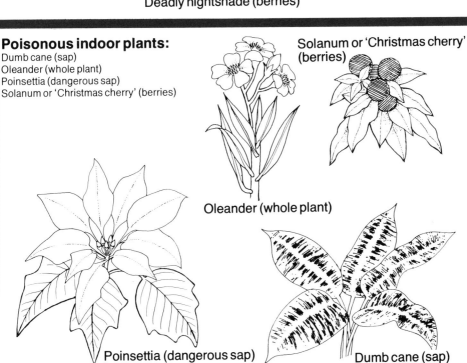

Solanum or 'Christmas cherry' (berries)

Oleander (whole plant)

Poinsettia (dangerous sap)

Dumb cane (sap)

68 Poisoning

Agricultural poisons absorbed through the skin:

There are so many chemicals used today in agriculture that it is difficult to generalise about them. The disturbing thing is that many of them are now available for the domestic market and so can present as a hazard even if you live in a town. As the symptoms are so variable it makes sense to say:

If you ever get any strange feelings after using pesticides, weedkillers or fertilisers, don't neglect them. Early, vague symptoms can quickly change into serious ones, so don't delay.

Some of these poisons affect breathing, others nerve conduction and many are absorbed through the skin or the lungs.

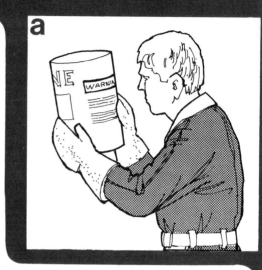

What to do:

1 Stop the person using the chemical.
2 Remove him gently from the area.
3 Remove contaminated clothing.
4 Wash exposed areas of the skin (preferably using rubber gloves yourself).
5 Give artificial respiration if breathing has stopped.
6 a Look at the container for suggested remedies. As a precaution, wear gloves when handling the chemical container and send it to the hospital with the person.
7 If the victim is sweating a lot and is hot, fan him and sponge with tepid water.

Poisoning by gas or smoke:

Although industrial gases and vapours of various kinds are encountered by those working with them, the gas most of us come across is domestic gas.

Although town gas used to be poisonous, natural gas which is supplied today, is not. It has a smell put into it so that leaks can be detected but the gas itself is not harmful.

However, it is still possible to be killed by gas because if a person is trapped in an air-tight room, the gas displaces the oxygen (which he is also using up as he breathes) and the person suffocates. Also, if an appliance is not burning properly, poisonous carbon monoxide may be produced.

The same happens with smoke but smoke has the additional disadvantage of actually damaging the lungs.

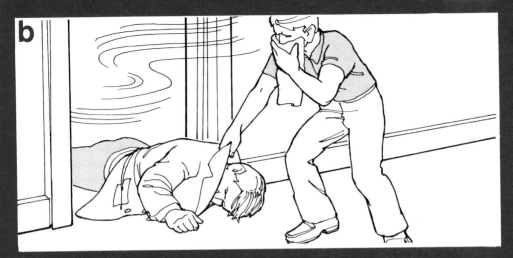

If you find someone in a gas or smoke-filled room:

1 Take a few deep breaths before entering.

2 Go in quickly, holding your breath and lift the victim to safety.

3 If you cannot remove him for any reason, throw open all the doors and windows, turn off the gas, leave and go back in as soon as the gas has dispersed. Do not do this if the place is on fire as it could draw the fire to the victim.

4 b If the room is filled with smoke, a wet cloth or towel wrapped across your mouth and nose may help to keep a little of the smoke out of your lungs. Keep low and if you cannot lift or drag the person clear, get help.

5 Ask someone else to go for help.

6 Give artificial respiration if necessary.

7 If the person is overcome by exhaust fumes in a closed garage, open doors, switch off the engine and proceed as above.

Prevention note

1 Have all gas appliances serviced regularly (at least once a year).

2 Never meddle with appliances yourself.

3 Never block up ventilators— natural gas burns safely with plenty of air but produces poisonous carbon monoxide if it has too little air.

4 Never leave the car engine running in a closed garage—the poisonous carbon monoxide in the exhaust can overcome you quicker than you think.

Around 1,000 people each day are involved in car crashes in the UK. Car accidents account for one third of deaths from all injuries and unusually for a serious medical situation, the public arrives before the professionals.

What to do:

1 Send someone for an ambulance unless the crash looks trivial and no one is injured.
He should tell
i The exact location of the accident;
ii how many cars are involved;
iii how many people seem to be injured;
iv if he thinks there are people trapped that could only be freed with lifting and cutting equipment;
v if there is any suggestion of fire/smouldering etc.
2 Make the scene safe by getting someone to stop traffic and by putting out warning triangles etc.
3 Park your car on the verge in such a way as to be able to illuminate the accident scene with your lights.
4 Stop people smoking.
5 Turn all the crashed cars' lights off, switch off the ignitions and apply the handbrakes.
6 Extinguish fire if you can. If not, get people clear.
7 Inspect the victims quickly and ask if they are all there.
8 If a person has been thrown out of a car, get someone to look for him and report back.

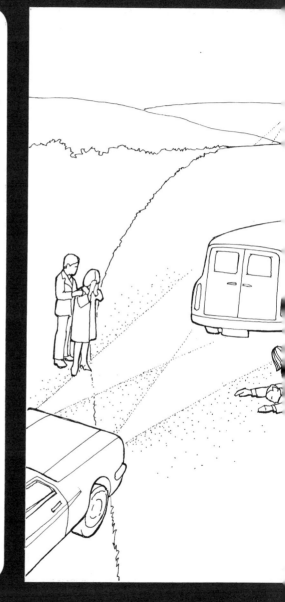

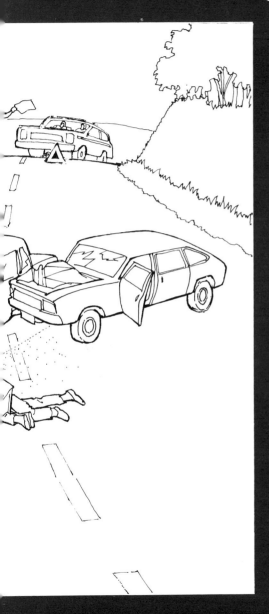

9 Deal first with any victims who are not breathing (page 20), who are bleeding seriously (page 28), or who have no pulse (page 24). **THESE ARE ABSOLUTELY LIFE-SAVING PRIORITIES.**
But do other things above first or you might all be killed or injured by other cars.

10 Remove those occupants who can easily get out.

11 Do **not** remove anyone who has signs of a broken back or neck unless there is a fire hazard or you cannot resuscitate him where he is. Leave the moving of injured people to the experts—you may do more harm than good.

12 While waiting for the emergency services, watch all the casualties and get others to help look after them.

13 Never let people wander off into nearby homes so that they can't be found by the emergency personnel. Prevent well-intentioned people from fiddling with and fussing around the casualties. The most difficult thing in an emergency is to do nothing and that is very often exactly what is called for.

14 Never try to lift a car off somebody unless there are at least two of you because you might drop it on the casualty and injure him further.

15 If someone is trapped by his seat belt and you can't see how it unlocks or if it is jammed—cut it. A seatbelt has to be replaced after a crash anyway, so don't hesitate.

The Fire Brigade should be called for any fire, however small.

If fire breaks out:

At home
If the house catches fire:

1a Get everyone in the house to a safe place on the ground floor so that they can get out quickly and safely.

OR leave the house altogether, closing doors, windows, fan lights, etc so that draughts don't feed the fire.

2 Don't assume someone else has called the fire brigade—do it yourself.

3 Only when everyone is safe should you start to tackle the fire, but only if you can do so without taking personal risks.

4b Use your fire extinguisher if you have one.

5 Wait for the fire brigade.

If you are trapped by a fire:

1c Close the door of the room.

2d Block up the gap under the door with bedding, towels, clothes etc, wetted if possible.

3e Attract attention at the window by shouting or waving a highly coloured article outside.

4f Should the room fill with smoke, go to the window and lean out for fresh air. If you can't do this, lie flat on the floor face down until help arrives or the situation gets desperate.

5 Should the room begin to burn or you can't breathe because of the smoke, tie sheets or other strong material together, secure one end to a heavy piece of furniture and use this 'rope' to lower yourself from the window.

6 Never jump out of a window. Lower yourself until you are hanging by your hands from the window sill and then drop, but do this only if you a) you can land safely, preferably on grass or soil, or b) if things are really hopeless inside the building. Remember, many people injure themselves unnecessarily by panicking and jumping from a window when, for the sake of another minute's wait, they could have been saved by firemen.

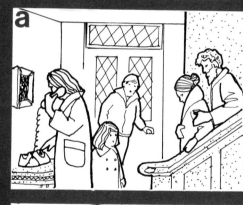

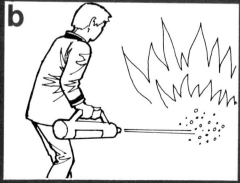

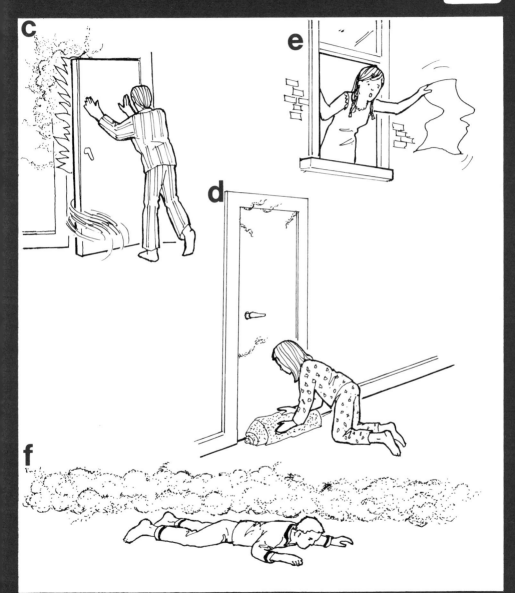

If someone's clothes catch fire:
1 If it's yourself—roll on the floor to smother the flames.
2a If it's someone else—get him to the ground by any means (push him over or trip him up if necessary). Throw a rug, blanket, coat, skirt etc over the burning area so as to exclude air from the flames. As you do this, protect the patient's face and yourself by using the coat or blanket as a shield.
3 If it's a child—stop him running around in panic (as this only fans the flames). Roll him in a blanket etc to put out the flames as above.

Smouldering clothes shouldn't be smothered because the hot fabric will be forced on to the patient's skin and so cause more damage. Carefully pull smouldering clothes off by unburnt parts. Put them in a fireproof bowl or other container or throw them on the floor and stamp on them. Call an ambulance. If the person is not seriously burnt, take him at once to a hospital.
NEVER TRY TO REMOVE CLOTHES THAT ARE CHARRED OR BURNT FIRMLY ON TO A PERSON. LEAVE THIS TO EXPERTS.

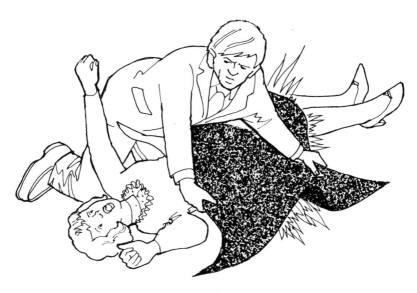

a

If a chimney catches fire:

1 Remove the hearth rug and anything around the hearth that might burn.
2b Gently splash water on to the fire in the grate. Do not flood the fire or the water will be thrown back at you as a cloud of scalding steam.
3 If you have a fine meshed fireguard, put it around the fire. If not, stand by with a bucket of water and a shovel to remove any burning soot that falls down the chimney and bounces back on to the carpet.

If a chip pan catches fire:

1 Turn off the heat (gas or electric).
2c Cover the pan with its lid, a tray or a damp towel. All of these starve the flames of air and so put them out.
DO NOT throw water on the pan or carry it to a sink or window. As you carry a burning pan, the flames are forced back on to you and your hand, making you drop the pan and spread the fire.

Fire extinguishers:

Every home should have a domestic fire extinguisher and preferably a fire blanket too. Make sure that these are kept in the hall or other easily accessible place. Don't keep them under the kitchen sink because there's a strong possibility that you won't be able to get to them in the event of a kitchen fire. Keep a check on the expiry date on extinguishers, they don't last for ever.

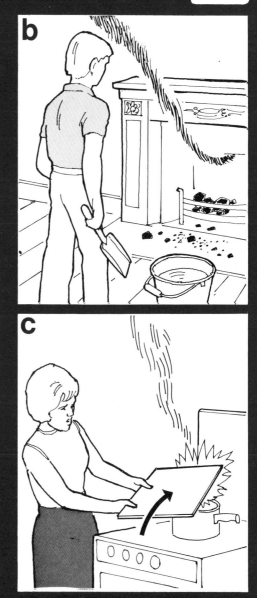

If a stove or heater catches fire:
1 Close the doors and windows in the room.
2 Smother the appliance with a heavy rug, towel, blanket etc.
3 Unless the fire goes out at once, get everyone out of the building.

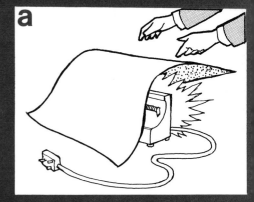

Electrical fires:
1 Switch off the source of the electricity supply and pull out the plug.
2a Smother the appliance with a heavy rug, towel, blanket etc.
3 Unless the fire goes out at once, get everyone out of the building.
4 NEVER THROW WATER ON TO AN ELECTRICAL APPLIANCE.

In the shed or garage:
1 Remove the car.
2 Remove any cans of petrol, cans of paint, creosote, etc.
3 Close all doors and windows.
4b Use a fire extinguisher if you have one.

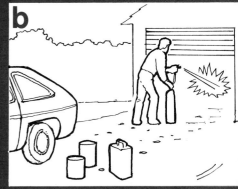

In a caravan:
1 Try simple measures to smother the fire or put it out with an extinguisher.
2 Turn off the gas cylinder outside and if possible disconnect it and roll it away.
3c Stand well clear.
4 Never leave children alone in a caravan.

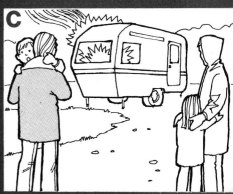

IF THE FIRE ISN'T IMMEDIATELY CONTROLLABLE, GET OUT OF THE VEHICLE QUICKLY AS FIRES SPREAD VERY RAPIDLY IN CARS AND CARAVANS.

In the car:
1 Stop the car.
2 Get everyone out.
3 Use a fire extinguisher if you have one and the fire is not too bad.
4d If engine compartment catches fire, open the bonnet a little only and push the nozzle of the fire extinguisher into the gap.
5e For a serious fire—stand well clear because the petrol tank may explode or poisonous fumes from burning plastics may harm your lungs.
6f If you see someone in a burning car, try to drag him free if you can do so without endangering yourself. Speedy action can prevent the inhalation of killer fumes. These are just as likely to kill as the flames.

REMEMBER THE FIRE BRIGADE SHOULD ALWAYS BE CALLED TO **ANY** FIRE HOWEVER SMALL.

BURNS: See page 56 for details.

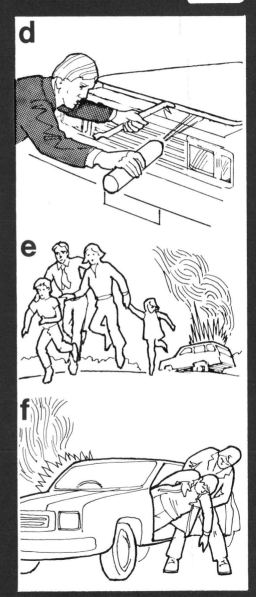

There are many causes of unconsciousness but you won't be able to sort them out. Leave the diagnosis to a doctor and in the meantime help the patient stay alive.

1 Make sure the person can breathe—before anything else.

2 Get someone to call an ambulance or doctor.

3 Suffocation is the greatest danger because the tongue can slip back and block the airway.

Wipe out any vomit, blood, food, false teeth etc with your fingers (inside a handkerchief if available).

4 If he isn't breathing, start resuscitation (page 20).

5 If he is breathing, lie him down in the recovery position, turn his head to one side and pull the jaw forward to clear the airway. If he makes gurgling or snoring noises you haven't cleared the airway.

6 Give nothing by mouth until the person himself can hold a cup and then he should only take tiny sips or he may vomit.

7 While awaiting professional help—stop bleeding (page 28) and prevent shock (page 34) if present.

8 Keep him in the recovery position and keep people away.

The Recovery position (a)

In many places in this book this position is mentioned. Many people have died unnecessarily because they have choked on their own tongue or vomit. This can be prevented by placing the person in the recovery position.

Always get an injured or unconscious person into this position as soon as possible **except** when you suspect a fracture, especially of the spine (see page 42) in which case DO NOT MOVE THE PERSON unless his life is threatened.

In such cases, stay by the head, turn it to one side and pull the chin forwards and upwards to clear the airway.

It is not easy to put someone into the recovery position if he is unconscious and much bigger than you so follow the technique described here and you won't hurt yourself or him.

1 Kneel beside the casualty as he lies on his back.

2 Put both arms by his sides.

3 Bring his far leg across his near one and pull his far hip over so that his far leg can rest on the ground near your knees. His thigh should be at right angles to his hip.

4 Take care of his head during all this (with your right hand) so that it doesn't roll on to the ground and hurt him.

5 Bring his far arm (which is now near your knees) up towards his face and use it to prop the body up a bit so he doesn't lie flat on his face. His upper arm should end up at right angles to the shoulder. His other arm is behind him, out straight, close to his body.

6 Adjust the position of the head so that the chin is pulled forwards and the head tilted backwards to clear the airway. Don't use pillows. If the person is on a bed or stretcher, raise its foot.

7 Do not leave him alone. Watch breathing and feel for the neck pulse from time to time. At any sign of either failing, resuscitate (page 20), start heart massage (page 24) or do both.

8 Look in his wallet to see if he carries a card or round his neck or wrist for a Medic-alert or Talisman medallion which might explain why he is unconscious. This could help in his later treatment.

9 Once you have done all this, provided the person is in no danger you can start enquiring as to the possible cause of the unconsciousness.

Head injuries are a common cause and must be taken seriously:

1 Any child who has been unconscious for however short a period must be seen by a doctor as soon as possible.

2 Anyone who has been 'knocked out' or suffered concussion should receive medical attention even if he feels all right. It is possible that there may be a fracture of the skull or other damage which isn't immediately apparent yet which might cause danger later. A person who has bruising around the eye sockets or watery or blood-stained fluid from the nose or ears must have immediate medical help.

3 Anyone who has speech or coordination problems after a period of unconsciousness must be seen by a doctor at once. Severe headache, dizziness, vomiting or double vision are other important warnings of possible complications.

a

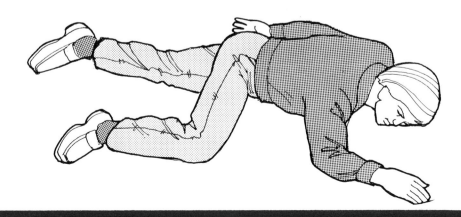

Don't
Use a tourniquet to stop bleeding—the chances are you'll do more harm than good by cutting off the blood supply for too long.

Don't
Throw the head back for a nose bleed—this makes the blood trickle to the back of the throat from where it is swallowed. Subsequent vomiting can make the nose bleed worse.

Don't
Give people salt water to make them sick when they swallow tablets. Don't give any water because rather than diluting the poison, water speeds up its absorption in the stomach.

Don't
Use antiseptics undiluted—they are no more effective than in the correct dilution and can damage the body.

Don't
Force a damaged elbow into a sling—you may do serious damage to the nerves and blood vessels nearby.

Don't
Force a zip fastener open if the foreskin is caught. Cut the bottom of the zip open and peel open the teeth of the zip from below.

Don't
Try to remove beads or other foreign bodies from children's ears and noses—leave them to the experts.

Don't
Leave hand injuries hanging down—keep them up to stop swelling. Pin the cuff to the person's lapel or dress high up on the chest.

Don't
Cover wounds or infections of the fingers with nylon finger stalls for more than an hour or so. The warm, moist conditions favour the breeding of germs.

Don't
Use other people's medicines.

Don't
Give anything by mouth to someone you suspect has broken a bone—he may need an anaesthetic later.

Don't
Make an emergency pillow for someone who has collapsed in the street—you may endanger his breathing by bending the neck forwards.

Don't
Leave an unconscious person for longer than it takes to summon help.

Don't
Move anyone you think has damaged his back unless he is threatened by danger.

Don't
Give unconscious people anything to drink or eat. Wait until the person is alert enough to hold a cup for **himself**.

Don't
Remove people from the scene of the crash because the ambulance crew may never find them.

Don't
Take people to hospital by private car after a serious accident or illness because you deprive them of the treatment they would receive in the ambulance.

Don't
Try lifting a vehicle off someone—you'll probably hurt yourself or fail and let it drop back on the person, so inflicting even more damage.

Don't
Touch anything until the mains supply has been switched off when you arrive at the scene of an electric shock.

Don't
Cover people up more when they have a fever.

This section of the book is not meant to be a medical encyclopaedia, nor a way of making the reader into a professor of medicine overnight! The subjects covered are basically those which, whilst not life-threatening, can be distressing, painful or simply worrying until you can get medical help. If you suffer from longstanding arthritis or bad breath, the chances are that you will have to come to terms with it, find a satisfactory treatment or at least be prepared to seek 'non urgent' medical advice. All the conditions covered here are sufficiently worrying in the short term to constitute an emergency—but not in the usually accepted sense of the word. If an epileptic friend has a simple fit, for example, it would be reassuring to know what to do (and what not to do), then you wouldn't panic.

As with the rest of the book, this section is not meant to replace medical advice from your doctor but should enable you to do **something** useful while you're waiting for the doctor to visit or for an appointment at the hospital and may even prevent you going to the local casualty department with something you could treat yourself.

If you are in any serious doubt about any condition—call your doctor. Don't use this section to outwit, out-diagnose or replace him. Having said this though, it's the responsibility of each of us to do what we can to help ourselves and our families. If we all insisted on medical care for all of the things in this section, every time we had them, doctors would be completely overwhelmed. Drawing the line is always difficult but the following pages give you guidance on this too.

Contents

Numbers given in blue refer to 'Useful Addresses' on pages 112 and 113.

A

Abscess

A bad spot or boil containing pus anywhere on the body. The treatment for any collection of pus is to let it out. Nature will do this eventually but in the meantime it can be painful and inconvenient to wait. If the abscess is on the face or hands it can be dangerous as well as painful. Always get medical help early for abscesses in these areas and never interfere with them.

For other abscesses, draw the pus out by applying a hot water bottle to the area over a simple dressing and keep it covered afterwards with a fresh, dry dressing. Doctors always say you shouldn't squeeze a pimple but people do it every day and come to no harm. When there is a definite white or yellow 'head' to an abscess or boil you can squeeze it after washing your hands thoroughly. Never squeeze so hard as to damage the surrounding skin and if the head doesn't come out easily, stop, wait another day and try again if necessary.

Never dig around with a needle, penknife or similar instrument. If the pus won't come out on its own, see a doctor.

Never use waterproof dressings such as nylon finger stalls or occlusive adhesive dressings because the bacteria in the abscess grow especially well under such wet, warm conditions and can spread to cause a wider and more serious infection of the tissues around the boil.

If you think the boil is spreading or if you notice any thin red lines in the skin surrounding an abscess, get medical help.

Always seek medical help for any abscess that is interfering with the use of a joint.

Never take the odd couple of antibiotic capsules or tablets that you happen to have in the medicine chest as this can lead to half treated infections that never properly clear up. If you need antibiotics, your doctor will prescribe a proper course. Badly and half treated abscesses can readily be troublesome for a very long time. If you take a few left over tablets or stop a proper course early, you may permit the infection to flare up again and it may not respond to that medicine the second time around.

Alcoholism 2, 3, 34

This is a complex disease that is almost impossible to treat at home. If a member of your family is an alcoholic you'll need help in order to lead a normal family life. Because alcoholism is a 'family disease' it has insidious effects which can be damaging to any or all of the family. If you have a problem like this, contact *Al-Anon Family Groups* (2).

If you are worried about your own drinking and want to get help, contact *Alcoholics Anonymous* (3). This organisation has 21,000 groups in 92 countries and has a vast experience of helping alcoholics.

Angina 14

A severe pain in the chest, arms or neck caused by starvation of blood to the heart muscle. Treating angina is often easy because the person who suffers from it has usually been told what to do by his doctor when the diagnosis was first made.

The problem with treating angina at home is that it is difficult (if not impossible) to distinguish between a really bad angina pain and a heart attack. Even doctors cannot always tell the difference without doing an electrocardiograph test. If someone has angina, sit him in a reclining position or lie him down; loosen any tight clothes; keep calm and help him to take one of his heart tablets (the TNT, trinitrin or glyceryl trinitrate type, NOT other heart tablets). If the pain doesn't go within half an hour, or if he becomes ill, call a doctor.

The person who has the angina is usually the best judge of how he feels. If he's really ill with an episode, you'll have to take over. Get an ambulance if 1) he stops breathing or his pulse stops (see pages 20 and 24 for emergency action); 2) he goes very pale, sweaty or even blue; 3) he loses consciousness; 4) the pain goes on for more than half an hour after taking the angina tablets; or 5) he becomes very distressed.

Should it be necessary to call for an ambulance, tell the ambulance officer as much as you can about the person's angina because in some areas there are specialised cardiac ambulances that they can send out. Simply saying 'Dad's collapsed on the sofa' tells them nothing.

Arthritis 12

Pain in a joint or joints. What you do depends on whether the pain has come on suddenly 'out of the blue' or has been with you for some time. Longterm pain in the joints doesn't call for emergency action but a painful, swollen joint of sudden onset can be very distressing.

Rest the part involved, take pain killing tablets, apply heat to the area and see your doctor as soon as you can.

Asthma 5, 14, 15, 32

Asthma is a condition affecting children and adults that makes them prone to attacks of wheezing and breathlessness. The airways of asthma sufferers are over-sensitive to certain provoking factors and react by narrowing and tightening up. This tightening up makes breathing difficult and can be very frightening to the asthmatic and those around him.

Most asthmatic children have allergies which bring on the attacks but emotional upsets, temperature changes, pollution, exercise and infection can also bring on attacks. By far the commonest allergy is to domestic house dust—specifically to the house dust mite. Children may also be allergic to grass pollen, pets, feathers in pillows, mould, foods and many other things.

Prevention is the best cure. Avoidance of any known allergic substances is the most obvious starting point but this can be difficult in practice. Drugs help greatly to prevent attacks and some children can be adequately protected against certain allergies by having a course of desensitising injections. A happy and relaxed family atmosphere and parents who understand the disease make a real difference to the number of attacks a child has.

Most parents get to know when their child is about to have an attack because he becomes pale and lethargic, coughs and has a running nose. If you have any prescribed drugs, use them at this stage and you may abort an attack.

Never panic. Although the sight of your child fighting for his breath may upset you, don't convey your alarm to him because this will make him worse. Whether the asthmatic is a child or an adult, keep calm, give him something to do, let in some fresh air and loosen any tight clothing.

There are four positions in which your child might be more comfortable—see which suits him best during an attack. 1) Lying on one side, slightly rolled forward with the knees bent. The top leg should be in front of the one underneath; 2) lying on one side as in 1) but on a slope of three or four pillows with an extra pillow filling in the gap between waist and armpit; 3) sitting or kneeling, forwards against a chair, with the upper chest supported by pillows and the back straight; or 4) sitting, leaning forward with a straight back, arms resting on thighs.

Get your child into one of these positions and get him to do diaphragmatic breathing (breathing from waist level rather than from the chest). He'll need to be taught this by his doctor or physiotherapist. It's worth practising the breathing with your child every day so that when he has an attack it'll seem natural to him to breathe this way.

Should your child not respond to these simple measures, call your doctor. Don't let the situation get desperate because it will then be much more difficult to treat. A very bad attack may mean the child will have to go into hospital.

B

Baby battering 31, 39, 40, 48

Many more mothers occasionally feel like harming their babies than is generally realised. Even the well-balanced, usually loving mother can feel like lashing out at her baby when she's overtired or stressed by poor domestic surroundings or other problems.

If you ever feel exasperated to the point of hurting your baby, don't wait until you're desperate but get another member of the family to look after the baby or call a friend or neighbour to help. When you're in this state, you and the baby alone are a bad combination. If you can't easily get any help, call the *Samaritans* as a last resort but try your doctor or health visitor first (see numbers in front of book). You may not want to involve 'professionals' because you fear they'll blame you for feeling the way you do about your baby, but they won't. Most professionals are understanding and used to dealing with this situation and certainly won't take the baby away from you unless absolutely necessary for your sake and the baby's sake. Once the immediate crisis is over, see your doctor or health visitor and try to sort out the underlying troubles that made you want to harm your baby in the first place. You will find the solution more readily with skilled help.

Blisters

These are produced by burns or by repeated rubbing and chafing of an area of skin. Under normal conditions, *don't burst blisters* because doing so increases the risk of infection. Simply cover them with sterile dry dressings and leave them. However, should the blister be so awkward because of its position that it causes a restriction of movement and function, prick it carefully as follows. Wash the blister itself with antiseptic solution, sterilise a large needle by boiling it or passing it through a flame until red hot, keep the needle away from anything else while it cools, pierce the blister in two places at the base and absorb the fluid that emerges on clean new cotton wool or gauze. Cover the whole area with a dry dressing until healed.

Breast abscess 4, 25, 33

Nearly ten per cent of breast feeding mothers suffer from a breast abscess in the weeks after childbirth. These abscesses are almost entirely preventable in the first place and arise only because we in the West feed our babies in such a strange way. Because we breast feed by the clock (if indeed we breast feed at all), the breasts become engorged (swollen) and the pressure within the breasts can block a milk duct. The blocked duct shows as a red, hot, tender lump in the breast and this often makes the woman feel shivery or 'flu-like.

First aid measures include feeding the baby much more frequently (to empty the breast); not limiting the length of feeds; massaging the lump gently but firmly towards the nipple; ensuring that your bra doesn't press on any particular area of the breast; varying the position in which the baby feeds at each feed and even during a feed; and using hot or cold compresses (whichever gives best relief). Antibiotics will only be necessary if all these methods have not dispersed the lump within 24 hours.

If a blocked duct is caught early, it will not go on to become infected and form a proper abscess (a walled-off, pus-filled structure within the breast). Once an abscess does form though it will probably (like abscesses elsewhere) need to be incised by a doctor to allow the pus to escape. If you have a breast abscess you should not feed the baby from that breast but continue to feed from the other one. Once the abscess has cleared up you can feed again from both breasts. In the meantime, express milk from the affected breast frequently and discard it. It may be possible to avoid incision by catching the abscess early and treating it with antibiotics. Your doctor will prescribe a suitable drug should it be indicated.

Breast lump 13, 26, 54

Lumps in the breast are fairly common and are most often nothing to do with cancer. But with one woman in twenty dying of breast cancer in the UK today, breast lumps must be taken seriously.

If you feel a lump, go to your doctor within 24 hours or to the first surgery on Monday if you find the lump over the weekend. He will feel it and tell you if he thinks it feels like a 'normal' lump that many women have in their breasts or if he thinks it needs a specialist opinion. Any breast lump associated with a recent (as opposed to a longstanding) inturning of the nipple or bleeding from the nipple must be seen by a doctor without delay.

One of the ways of saving yourself a lot of worry is to get into the habit of examining your breasts regularly every month. Do this after your period and get used to the feel of your breasts so that you'll pick up a lump early on, should one occur. Early treatment makes a difference to the outcome. **Don't delay going to your doctor because you're afraid**. Delay can only make things worse.

Bronchitis

An inflammation of the large air tubes in the chest. There are two different conditions covered by this term and they need different treatment. Acute bronchitis comes on after 'flu and colds and produces a dry, painful cough and tightness in the chest. Later on, yellow, brown or green phlegm may be coughed up. The best treatment for this condition is to keep the room air moist by having a kettle steaming away in a corner. Coupled with steam inhalations (available from chemists) this can reduce chest tightness and help bring up the phlegm. Hot drinks also help bring up the phlegm. Most people get better but some will need antibiotics. If you bring up yellow, brown or green phlegm, tell your doctor. Antibiotics may not be necessary.

Chronic bronchitis is a long term illness seen in cigarette smokers and those who have lived in polluted air. These people will know they are 'bronchitics' and should have been told that there is no cure. The condition can be prevented from getting worse by 1) stopping smoking; 2) moving away from polluted air; 3) losing weight; 4) getting medical treatment for even trivial chest infections; and 5) doing regular breathing exercises.

C

Car sick children

1) If you talk about the subject in front of or to your children, they're more likely to be sick; 2) if your child does tend to be sick, treat the subject lightly and don't make an invalid of him; 3) keep to light, easily digestable meals before travelling; 4) have a strong brown paper bag ready (but not obviously so); 5) keep a car window open a little, close to the child; 6) keep the children occupied with games, stories or tapes on the car cassette player, if you have one; and 7) ask Dad not to drive too fast and to stop regularly for short breaks. If none of these measures works, get help from you doctor.

Colds

There is no cure for the common cold but the symptoms of headache, runny nose, fever, aches, pains and weakness are worth treating. The best treatment for a cold is still bed rest. A day in bed does more good than anything else. Take aspirin in the recommended dose for a headache or fever; drink plenty of fluids; and take 1 g of Vitamin C twice a day (it may do some good and will do no harm). If you're going to use nasal decongestants to help you breathe more easily, follow the instructions carefully—never overdo them.

If you get breathless or cough up green or yellow phlegm, seek medical help.

Colic 33

An intermittent pain caused by the contraction of a hollow organ or tube in the body. In adults, colic is typically caused by gall stones or kidney stones but most of us have suffered from abdominal pains that 'come and go' at some time, without having stones. The cause of these pains is hardly ever found but the condition often improves once the person has had his bowels open. Any severe pain that comes and goes and is bad enough to make you feel sick or put you to bed must be assessed by a doctor. While waiting for the doctor, apply gentle warmth to your abdomen.

In children, 'three month' or evening colic is a term used to explain the screaming sessions that occur usually in the early evenings up to the age of about three months. The usual remedies of food, comfort, drink and nappy change seem to make little difference. A baby may cry at this time of day because of tension (mother is getting tired and is especially busy) or boredom (because he's been sleeping and eating all day and is ready to be amused).

If you are breast feeding, let your baby suck on and off all evening on your lap, if necessary. Cut out all cows' milk and milk products from your diet for a few days because some babies get colic from the traces of cows' milk in their mother's breast milk.

Colic in babies is in most cases no longer thought to be due to 'wind'. Anti-colic medicines are of little help and your baby will benefit most from being carried around (perhaps in a sling) and comforted.

Conjunctivitis 21

An inflammation of the membrane covering the eye. Usually caused by bacteria, it can be secondary to grit or even trauma. The eye becomes pink and the eyelashes stick together with yellow discharge, especially on first waking. Bathe the eye with boric acid solution several times a day and tell your doctor as soon as practicable. He will give you drugs or an ointment which cure the condition very quickly. Don't share face flannels or towels whilst you have this condition as it is easy to pass on. Wash your hands after touching your eyes and change your pillowslip daily.

Contraceptive failure 22, 35

There are three crises that can occur with contraceptives. The first is forgetting the Pill, the second is the failure of a barrier method and the third, the falling out of your coil (IUD).

Pill failure is relatively common because unless you're absolutely rigid about when you take it each day, it's easy to forget. If you discover that you've forgotten a pill within 24 hours of when you should have taken it, take another immediately and then take the next one at the normal time.

If you discover your mistake between 24–48 hours after you should have taken a pill, take two pills together immediately and then catch up with your old routine.

For any gap of more than 48 hours, take two pills per 24 hours until you've made up the deficit and are back on schedule again as judged by taking the right pill on the right day marked on the pack. In this case you should also use another method such as a diaphragm or a sheath together with contraceptive jelly to be sure you're safe. Your next cycle should see you back to normal again, so don't worry.

Should your IUD (coil or loop) fall out, there's nothing you can do yourself, so simply tell the doctor or clinic that fitted it and go and have it replaced as soon as you can. You are not protected at all, of course, while it is out, so use some other method in the meantime.

If a sheath bursts or comes off while the penis is in the vagina, if you find your diaphragm has a hole in it or if you think you may have got some sperms in your vagina during the withdrawal method, you can do one of two things. First, you can go to certain family planning clinics or hospital specialist clinics for a 'morning after' pill (you'll need to phone around a bit to find one that offers it) or you can do something at once for yourself at home. 1) make up a solution of vinegar and water (half and half) and crouching over a bowl in the bath, splash the liquid up into your vagina vigorously; 2) using the vinegar and water mixture, thoroughly soak a tampon and push it high up into your vagina. A combination of 1 and 2 is a good idea. Neither of these methods is foolproof, of course, but they're worth trying and may be better than doing nothing.

Lastly, don't panic if you think you have a contraceptive failure. Bear in mind that except for the days around the middle of your cycle you're most unlikely to conceive anyway and that might put your mind at rest.

Coughing

If someone is coughing severely try to find out if he has inhaled something that might be choking him. If he tells you or signals that he has, see Choking page 50. Otherwise, if the cough is severe, sit the person down, reassure him and keep calm. A sharp pat or two on the back between the shoulder blades may dislodge a plug of sticky mucus that's provoking the coughing. Any cough that is present for more than two weeks or any cough that makes the person bring up coloured phlegm must be investigated by a doctor. **Never ignore a persistent cough.**

Dry coughs serve no purpose and annoy the rest of the household, especially at night. If the back of the throat is especially sensitive (after 'flu, for example) proprietary tablets and hot drinks can be used with effect. Linctus or cough medicine may also be useful for this sort of cough. A teaspoonful of honey may also give enough relief to enable you to drop off to sleep.

Should a dry cough become productive (make you bring up phlegm), keep warm, try inhalations, have a kettle boiling in the corner of your room to moisten the air and take medicine designed to bring up the loosened phlegm (your doctor will prescribe you this).

Whooping cough in children is characterised by severe bouts of coughing in which the child becomes very distressed, may go blue and vomits. It is a serious disease, so if your baby or child ever coughs severely and repeatedly (with or without the classical 'whoop' as he breathes in) phone your doctor. Keep the child warm and **keep calm.** Cuddle him up close to you and reassure him. After a bout of coughing, give him some food and drink in the hope that he'll manage to digest it before the next bout of coughing. Give him lots of small meals rather than a few big ones. Have a kettle boiling in the child's room until he goes to sleep. In really severe cases you can even make your own steam tent under a sheet but **take care with the boiling water.** Cough mixtures are useless for whooping cough—leave them alone.

Croup 32

A type of laryngitis (inflammation of the vocal cords) in children that makes breathing difficult and distresses both child and parents. Every breath is accompanied by a high-pitched croaking or crowing noise. Croup is usually caused by a virus and therefore cannot be treated with antibiotics. It can also be caused by whooping cough, diphtheria and foreign bodies in the voice box.

Call your doctor if 1) your baby has any difficulty breathing or 2) there is any pulling-in of the lower end of the breastbone and side ribs with each breath.

You can do a lot to help. 1) Reassure your child—fear and tension make the croup worse; 2) keep calm yourself or your alarm will spread to him; and 3) get an electric kettle boiling away in a safe corner of the room—the moist air helps the breathing. If these remedies don't work, the doctor may advise treatment in hospital.

Cystitis 53

An inflammation of the bladder caused by bacterial infection. It occurs at any age and in both sexes but is very much more common in women.

Cystitis is characterised by pain in the lower abdomen and sometimes between the legs; a frequent desire to pass urine (even immediately after the bladder has been emptied); burning pain in the urinary passage as urine is passed; sometimes pain in the small of the back (one side or both); sometimes fever; and the urine may look normal, cloudy or bloody.

Even quite severe cystitis may not make the woman feel generally ill. Having said this, the pains can be so agonising that first aid action is necessary even before medical help is sought.

Cystitis always warrants medical investigation and treatment the first time it happens. Many women though learn to live with their cystitis, can prevent attacks completely, or simply deal with them at home without going on to antibiotics. While waiting for medical attention there are several things that can be done.

1 Take 2 tablets of any of the commonly used painkillers.
2 Drink 150 ml ($\frac{1}{4}$ pint) of barley water or plain water every 20 minutes until the attack is over. This produces the fluid you need to flush the infection out of your bladder.
3 Over a 2 hour period, take 3 doses of 1 level teaspoonful of bicarbonate of soda dissolved in a glass of warm water. This alters the acidity of the urine and makes it more difficult for the bacteria to survive.
4 Drink plenty of black coffee. This stimulates the kidneys to produce large quantities of dilute urine.
5 Fill 2 hot water bottles, wrap them in towels so that you don't burn yourself and place one on your back and one between your legs up against your lower abdomen.
6 Every time you pass urine, wash the area well but gently with warm water, dabbing dry rather than scrubbing with the towel.
7 Stay in bed if you can while the attack lasts.
8 Get help from your doctor.

D

Despair 18, 30, 48

Most of us feel desperate at some time in our lives. Bereavement, divorce, loss of a boyfriend, girlfriend or parents, redundancy or even depression can reduce the strongest and most normal of us to despair.

If you feel like this, talk to someone. Get a friend to come round, talk to a neighbour or relative, or, in the last resort, call the *Samaritans* (look under *Samaritans* in the phone book). They are used to listening to people in this situation and are a great help in the crisis stage. You can also phone the police or the Social Services Department at your local town hall (look under Social Services in the front of your phone book). These departments have emergency services 24 hours a day.

Cruse clubs (17) specialise in helping the bereaved; Depressives Anonymous (18) will help if you are depressed; and Family Service Units (look under this title in the phone book) are a great help too in a variety of desperate situations. If your child has died, the *Compassionate Friends* (16) will help.

Don't wait until things get so bad that you can't cope—get help early.

Diabetes 7

A disease of unknown cause that results from the person having too little insulin in his bloodstream. About three quarters of all diabetics can be controlled with diet and tablets alone but the other one quarter has to take insulin for the rest of their lives.

Should you run out of insulin, your nearest hospital casualty department or chemist will give you a supply in an emergency.

Diabetics can become very ill if they get the balance of insulin, exercise and food intake wrong. Almost always the trouble they get into is caused by too low a blood sugar. Should a diabetic exhibit a combination of the following signs, he'll know that he needs sugar by mouth to make him better. Sometimes though the very condition itself makes him confused and in severe cases unconscious, so your prompt action could save his life. Signs to look for are; sweating, trembling, tingling around the tongue and lips, weakness, palpitation, hunger with nausea, staggering as if drunk,

uncharacteristic behaviour, bad temper and yawning.

Most diabetics carry some sugar lumps in their pockets or handbag for just such an emergency, so ask if he has something (assuming of course that the person is conscious and rational). If he is conscious, help him to eat a couple of sugar lumps or a teaspoonful of jam. **Never force an unconscious diabetic to eat or drink anything**. Only give him sweet drinks or food when he is sufficently recovered to sit up and hold the cup or glass himself.

If he is unconscious and so cannot take anything by mouth, call an ambulance. Whenever you find anyone who is unconscious, look through his pockets or handbag for lumps of sugar or a diabetic card and if found, this will give you and medical helpers the answer to the cause of the unconsciousness.

Once you have given the first sweet food or drink, stay with the person and give him more if he doesn't seem to be improved within two to three minutes.

Should anyone you know who is a diabetic seem to be drunk, think twice! Further information about diabetes can be obtained from the *British Diabetic Association.* (7).

Double vision 21

A serious symptom that needs medical attention. It may be caused by simple astigmatism (which can be corrected by glasses); a slipped lens in the eye; incipient cataract; or by an imbalance in the muscles that control eye movements. To discover which eye is affected, cover up one eye at a time and then wear a patch of something over the offending eye while you go to see your doctor.

Double vision isn't dangerous in itself but can be very distressing and even hazardous if you're driving or operating machinery. Covering up the affected eye will enable you to see normally until the condition can be cured but NOT well enough to drive or operate machinery!

Dysentery

An avoidable infectious illness caused by swallowing dysentery germs. These get into the mouth on unwashed hands, contaminated food and drink or on objects such as toys, cutlery or pencils which have been touched by an infected person. The swallowed germs breed in the bowel and cause diarrhoea, tummy pains, vomiting and fever. If anyone in your household or at work gets an illness that's like this they should see a doctor. Should the illness turn out to be dysentery, the doctor is bound to tell the Community Physician, whose job it is to prevent the infection spreading to others.

If you have someone with dysentery in the house you must wash your hands with soap under running water before preparing food or drink, before handling the baby and before leaving the home. You must also wash your hands after using or cleaning the lavatory; after doing anything with or to the ill person; after changing the baby's nappy or after washing clothes or sheets. Don't share towels—use paper tissues or towels if possible and destroy these by burning.

Food. Always wash your hands before and after handling food. Serve the food hot and then store it in a refrigerator. Keep friends and visitors away while the person is still ill. Store your pets' food separately from yours.

Laundry. Put all the infected person's dirty laundry into a plastic bin or bag apart from all the rest of the family's wash and do not wash it by hand. If you have a machine, set it to the hottest setting or otherwise boil the laundry. This can be difficult but do not take things to the launderette or send them to the laundry as this will spread the infection. If you haven't a washing machine and can't boil the laundry, tell your local health department which will supply you with a special disinfectant in which you can steep the soiled things.

Lavatory. Wash your hands after using the lavatory. When cleaning the lavatory use rubber gloves which should be kept in the lavatory for this purpose only—don't do the washing up with them on! After each person has used the lavatory, the door handle, flush handle or knob and lavatory seat must be cleaned with a scouring powder containing bleach or a disinfectant.

Dysentery is a serious, yet preventable disease. If you take care, you can save others a lot of worry, illness and trouble.

E

Earache

A common and very unpleasant condition in children but rare in adults. It is usually caused by bacteria spreading up from the nose and throat via the tube that connects these areas to the ear. The child often has a cold for a few days before the earache. The pain of earache may be very severe and may be accompanied by a fever of over 38°C (100°F).

Should your child show any signs of earache (such as pulling on the ear) or if he has unexplained fever, vomiting, diarrhoea or loss of appetite, he may have a middle ear infection (otitis media). Your doctor may prescribe antibiotics and possibly nose drops too but there are additional things you can do both before and after you have seen him. Give the child a full dose of aspirin (as directed for his age on the pack) and hold a warm hot water bottle wrapped in a cloth against the affected ear. If he has a very high fever, keep him cool as described below under Fever.

Ear infections in children are serious; they need medical treatment and should not be ignored.

F

Fever

High body temperatures (fevers) are usually caused by bacterial or viral infections. How do you know if you or your child has a fever? The easiest way is to take his temperature with a domestic clinical thermometer. Learn how to use it if you have one so that you are confident when you tell your doctor over the phone what your child's temperature is. However, it is by no means essential to have a thermometer, as any parent will be able to tell if his child is hot to the touch, red, sweaty and feverish. Actual temperature readings are notoriously unhelpful in children because the temperature is a poor guide to how ill a child is. Your impression is much more important.

While you're waiting for the doctor to come, **don't** give any antibiotics you have lying around, simply cool the person down by 1) giving aspirin in the recommended dose for the age of the person, 2) turning off the heating in the room and removing some clothes and bedclothes, 3) sponging his body with tepid water and 4) giving iced drinks. **Always tepid sponge a child who has had a convulsion as a result of a fever.** Don't be afraid to get the child completely naked on the bed and sponge him down on a plastic or rubber sheet. There is far more danger in keeping a child too warm than in cooling him down when he has a fever. If your child has a febrile (fever) convulsion, tell your doctor at once or call an ambulance. Once you have tepid sponged him, wrap damp cloths loosely around his neck and groins and take his temperature every ten minutes. When his temperature falls to 38.5°C (101°F) cover him lightly with a sheet. If his temperature rises again, repeat the procedure.

Any adult who has a fever should rest in bed and take plenty of fluids by mouth. Eat according to how you feel and don't get up until your temperature is back to normal or until you feel quite well again. If you have repeated fevers, tell your doctor.

Fish hook in skin

Never attempt to tear a fish hook out of the skin as you'll simply rip the flesh on the barb.

Simply cut away the clothing around the hook, then cut off the line and lure.

Push the hook through the skin so that the point and barb emerge the other side and tape the hook flat to the skin. Get medical help. Really small hooks can be pushed through completely after cutting the line. If you do this, put a dab of antiseptic cream on the area and cover with a waterproof adhesive dressing. You should then have an anti-tetanus injection.

'Flu

A viral infection that you can carry around and spread without knowing it. The germs are spread in the air and can infect someone else in your company even if you don't cough over him. It's worth taking care by sneezing or coughing into a handerchief.

'Flu is characterised by aching limbs and back, shivering and a fever. Later, sweating may be profuse and your eyes may hurt as you move them. There is nothing a doctor can do that you cannot do yourself, so don't get your doctor in unless you have a history of chest trouble.

Go to bed at once, drink plenty of fluids 2–3½ litres (4–6 pints) a day for an adult, keep warm (but have some fresh air in the room) and take aspirin in the full recommended dose to bring down the fever and relieve the aches.

Keep people away, especially children and those with known chest diseases (such as bronchitis). Don't allow dirty handkerchieves to collect in the house when someone has 'flu. Either launder them as quickly as possible in a washing machine set at its hottest or boil them.

Better still, use disposable handkerchieves and flush them down the lavatory or burn them.

After 3 or 4 days, the worst of the symptoms will have gone but you may feel weak or depressed for weeks afterwards. If you are old or at special risk you should ask your doctor about an anti-'flu injection.

G

Gumboil

An abscess at the root of a tooth. This is usually a very unpleasant condition because not only is there pain in the gum but any pressure on, or even temperature change of the tooth produces pain. However, by the time the boil at the root of the tooth is at its worst the nerve will be dead and sensation therefore lost.

Superficial treatments are really not much help and the only useful thing is for your dentist to let the pus out. This is usually done by drilling up through the root of the tooth, so providing a canal down which the pus can flow. The canal is then plugged with a temporary, antiseptic filling.

Emergency dental care is extremely hard to come by in this country out of regular working hours and even fairly big hospitals can't do much to help. If severe, see your doctor who will probably recommend that you take penicillin and go to bed if you feel really bad. Contact your dentist as soon as you can. Local warmth over the area is soothing but there's little else you can do. Avoid very hot and cold foods, and alcohol.

H

Hallucinations 27, 30, 38, 44, 49

These are false perceptions which bear no reality to the real world. An illusion (such as a magician performs) is 'real' but is simply a sort of trick which fools the senses. Hallucinations are very different and much more serious because there is **no** base in reality for them. The sad thing is that the person who suffers from hallucinations believes that they are real and it is this belief in the face of evidence to the opposite that makes us define these people as seriously mentally ill. Any of the senses can be involved in hallucinations; voices may be heard, monsters or animals seen, gas smelt and so on. The vast majority of people who experience hallucinations are suffering from a serious mental condition called schizophrenia which is the commonest serious mental condition there is. It is seen mostly in young people under the age of 25 and fills about a fifth of all hospital beds. One person in a hundred is likely to suffer from schizophrenia.

As with many other mental illnesses, the people around a schizophrenic often fear that he will run amok or harm others. This is extremely unlikely but it's preferable to get medical help before things get anywhere near this bad. If a previously bright and normal adolescent becomes moody and spends lots of time alone in his room; becomes impossible to communicate with; has moods inappropriate to the situation; or can't think properly, get medical help—don't wait until he starts having hallucinations.

Normal people can experience hallucinations just as they are going off to sleep or during high fevers but if ever anyone has them at other times he should have medical help. Keep calm and don't get alarmed or angry with the person as he can't 'pull himself out of it'. To him the hallucinations are all too real and often terrifying. Get medical help at once. Some families fear going to a doctor because they think the affected person will be put into a mental hospital. However, mental hospitals are taking fewer people in and more mentally ill people are managing very well in the community than ever before.

Headache

Usually a trivial and short-lived symptom and very rarely a sign of serious disease. Most headaches are caused by anxiety or worry as the muscles of the scalp tense up. Migraine (see page 99) is a serious cause of headache that needs special treatment. Meningitis can cause headache but this is a rare condition. Should you ever have a headache which makes you vomit and produces a stiff neck, call the doctor at once. Eye strain, neck muscle strain, constipation and the hordes of other 'popular' causes of headache are probably not medically acceptable in the light of present knowledge.

If you have a headache, take a simple painkiller in the recommended dose, rest if it's really bad, or go for a walk if it is not. Recurrent headaches or those that come on first thing in the morning should be investigated by a doctor. If eating any particular food produces a headache—cut it out of your diet.

Heartburn

A burning sensation behind the lower end of the breast bone usually worst when lying down or bending down. People with a condition called hiatus hernia suffer from heartburn a lot as do some pregnant women. Many of us get it from time to time as a part of simple indigestion.

Short-lived heartburn can be treated with indigestion tablets or other alkaline 'tummy mixtures'. A glass of milk also helps.
Persistent heartburn needs medical investigation. If you are told you have a hiatus hernia, 1) lose weight; 2) avoid bending over to do up shoes etc; 3) sleep with the head of the bed raised on blocks; 4) use plenty of pillows; 5) stop smoking; 6) eat smaller meals; and 7) take the medicine prescribed.

If ever you get heartburn accompanied by pain in the arm or neck, see your doctor as soon as you can because a pain that is sometimes indistinguishable from heartburn can be angina or even a heart attack. Any heartburn that makes you feel really ill as opposed to simply uncomfortable needs medical attention.

Hiccough

A disturbance in the synchronous action of the lid that shuts off the upper end of the airway tube and the diaphragm muscle. The real fault is that the diaphragm contracts out of step. Most hiccoughs are caused by simple indigestion; hot spicy foods; exercise too soon after eating; or nervousness. There are a few more serious causes too.

Most hiccoughs go within an hour and traditional manoeuvres such as sipping water from the wrong side of a glass are as good as anything. Deep breathing, holding the breath or rebreathing air for a short time in a paper bag can all be tried but no one method seems best.

If hiccoughs go on for more than three hours, see a doctor.

Hysteria 30

A neurotic condition in which bodily signs and symptoms are present even though the person is in fact physically well. The hysterical personality is well recognised by doctors. Such people are dramatic, attention seekers and like creating scenes. They are emotionally shallow and insecure, sexually titillating but frigid deep down. They manipulate their families and friends and have learned, often during childhood, that sickness can be rewarding.

Hysterical fits can take the form of epilepsy-like attacks with strange noises and rolling on the ground but unlike the person with epileptic fits, the hysterical person will never hurt herself. Calm the woman down if she is like this but don't slap her face or shake her as this will do no good. Keep her under close supervision (which is what she wants) and then when it is all over, speak to her doctor about it and get his advice.

In a condition called conversion hysteria, the person's anxiety actually produces real physical debility such as true paralysis or blindness. This can be very distressing for those around and medical help is needed so that physical illness can be excluded with certainty. Don't panic though, especially if the person has had similar 'fits' before or is known to have a hysterical personality. Psychotherapy may be needed in the long term but while this is having an effect, the people around the hysteric will have to cope as calmly as possible with this distressing manifestation of anxiety neurosis.

I

Incontinence 20

A condition in which the sufferer is unable to hold his or her water (urine) and so wets himself either continuously or from time to time. Cystitis (see page 89) makes you want to pass water frequently but is not real incontinence. True incontinence is seen in stroke patients and people who have certain spinal injuries and nerve diseases. Stress incontinence (the involuntary passing of water on coughing and straining) may follow childbirth and if left untreated can become worse in later life. Severe constipation can cause dribbling in both sexes and an enlarged prostate gland in men can have the same effect. Some old people find they need to pass water very often and yet have difficulty in holding it until they get to the lavatory.

If you are incontinent, see your doctor as he may be able to help or may refer you to a specialist. If expert help is no use or if you are awaiting treatment, here are some

things you can do. 1) If your lavatory is a long way away, keep a bottle or commode handy. There are specially shaped containers for women and a hot water bottle can be useful as a last resort for men. 2) Wear clothes that are easy to get out of in a hurry. Women can wear knickers with loose elastic and men have their zip flies replaced with Velcro fastenings. 3) If stress incontinence occurs after childbirth, practice the exercises you are taught for several months. 4) Go to the lavatory much more frequently (every hour or two) even if you don't feel like it. 5) Don't reduce the amount you drink but don't drink too much after tea time.

If you still have problems in spite of all these precautions, ask your doctor to get you help from the social worker (who'll supply equipment, sanction alterations to your lavatory or arrange a home help) or district nurse (who can arrange bed protection, a special laundry service and disposable pads).

A Constant Attendance Allowance can be arranged if you need constant care during the day or night and if you are receiving Supplementary Benefit or Pension an additional allowance can be made for heating and extra laundry. Ask your local DHSS office about these. More information is available from the Incontinence Adviser, *Disabled Living Foundation* (20).

Insomnia

The inability to sleep. We all suffer from temporary or slight insomnia from time to time when we are stressed or worried but this type is often cured by small amounts of alcohol before retiring, by exercise, or by increased sexual activity.

For mild degrees of sleeplessness, try going through a regular routine every night. Hot baths and warm drinks or alcohol (especially in the old) are all good sleep producers. Some people find that something to eat or a walk before bed is helpful. Stop worrying about losing sleep—the worry will do you more harm than the sleep loss. Calm down before you go to bed, switch off the day's problems and lose yourself in a book or something else. Don't forget that we all need very different amounts of sleep. Don't worry because you seem to need so much less than your spouse—as long as you're fresh and happy during the day on the amount you get—so well and good.

Persistent insomnia is very troublesome because the person ends up very tired and depressed. Ironically, depression is one of the commonest causes of severe insomnia. The person wakes at 3 or 4 am or cannot go off to sleep at all. Treatment is essential for this condition. If you're on sleeping pills, 1) don't take them with alcohol; 2) only take the number directed; 3) keep them away from the bedside just in case you take another dose by mistake when you're half asleep; and 4) keep them away from children. Don't be ashamed of taking sleeping tablets but treat them for what they are—props to help you temporarily. Try to find out why you're not sleeping and cure that. It could be something as simple as a bad bed.

Itching

This can be a symptom of many conditions. Very commonly insects bite unknown to the person himself. Certain man-made fabrics increase the amount of sweat on the skin and this can cause itching. Allergies, eczema, nettlerash, sunburn and scabies are just a few of the many possible causes.

Many people wash too often and remove nature's fats from their skins and this may make the skin itch. The treatment here is to wash less frequently with soap.

Itching around the back passage or vagina must be investigated by a doctor (see also page 111).

Scratching is usually the best short term cure for itching from the sufferer's point of view but unfortunately tends to make the itching worse in the long term. Try to leave the skin alone or apply a cold cream or calamine lotion to the affected area. Should an itch go on for more than two days, see your doctor.

If you itch especially around your waist, between the thighs, between the finger knuckles or in your armpits, you may have scabies. See your doctor (see also page 122).

With care you can distinguish some of the common causes of itching yourself. Flea bites show as red spots scattered over the body; itchy allergic conditions usually present as raised, red, blotchy weals; head lice are confined to the scalp and nits can often be seen on the hairs; and fungal infections of the skin take the form of pink areas with distinctly defined red borders. If you think you have any of these, see your doctor.

J

Jaundice

Yellowness of the skin or the whites of the eyes caused by the deposition of bile pigments in the skin and eyes. This condition may be accompanied by fever, loss of appetite, diarrhoea and vomiting, pale putty-coloured stools, dark urine or itching.

Any yellowness must be assessed by a doctor who will find the cause and treat it. There is nothing you can do in the meantime.

L

Loneliness 18, 24, 29, 36, 37

This is often a long term problem but can be accentuated after a bereavement, after leaving home or after a domestic crisis of some kind. Loneliness is a serious social condition that needs just as careful handling as many medical diseases. After all, it can lead to depression or even suicide attempts.

Prevention is the best cure. Go to people who can help you. Talk to your general practitioner and get details of adult education courses in your area (your local town hall or library has lists of what's available). You may not think you want to learn anything but simply getting out to meet people for one or two nights a week will open your life up and at least enable you to meet people who share your interests.

Write to the *National Institute of Adult Education* (37) for ideas. There's nothing like helping other people to overcome your own loneliness. Enquire at your local hospital, WRVS, St John's or Red Cross. They all need help in one way or another and you'll enjoy being useful to others. There's a Voluntary Social Services Directory and Handbook available from the *National Council of Social Services* (36).

If you are separated, divorced or widowed, loneliness can be a real problem even if you still have children around you and you seem to be always busy. Consult the *National Association for the Divorced and Separated* (29); *The Cruse Club* Headquarters, (an organisation especially for the bereaved) (17); or the *Solo Clubs* (50).

Should you find yourself alone in a city, contact the *YWCA* or the *YMCA*. In London, *GALS (Girls Alone in London)* (24) can help. Young mothers are often very lonely especially in tower blocks or on new estates. The best way round this problem is to join local groups (mother and toddler clubs, church groups, WI, etc) and never miss an opportunity to get to know other young mothers at your local baby clinic.

Lumbago 6

A non-specific back condition including stiffness on waking; stiffness after unaccustomed exercise; difficulty rising from a chair; discomfort in sitting for long periods, especially on car journeys; inability to stand upright and any back pain limiting movement.

Lumbago is usually caused by muscle and ligament strains or even tears. In severe cases a disc may have partially slipped.

Most attacks cure themselves within two weeks but bed rest is useful in the meantime. Take painkillers and place a hot water bottle over the affected area. Gentle massage from a spouse can help and some people get relief from hanging by their hands from a door or beam.

If you are worried that this kind of backache isn't going as quickly as you think it should, see your doctor. If you get pins and needles, any other strange sensations or indeed any loss of sensation in your legs, or problems with passing urine, consult your doctor.

M

Migraine 9, 28

Not every bad headache is migraine. Migraine is a one-sided headache which is often very unpleasant. There is often a warning sensation beforehand which can be very varied and ranges from dizziness and feeling sick to visual disturbances and irritability. In some people certain things actually trigger the attack. Such triggers include television, flashing lights, flickering sunlight when driving past trees, alcohol and worry. Altogether there are about 20 or 30 trigger factors.

Although the features of migraine vary enormously from person to person and can even vary within any one person over a lifetime, most sufferers get used to the pattern of their own attacks and can help themselves to a certain extent. Migraine is a condition that needs professional medical diagnosis and treatment but once the

person has been sorted out medically he can usually help himself.

If you have been diagnosed as having migraine, 1) avoid trigger situations whenever possible; 2) always keep a small supply of your tablets, inhaler, suppositories or injections handy with you; 3) as soon as you suspect an attack is coming on, take your medication; 4) should you start an attack while driving, riding or operating any sort of machinery, **STOP**. Because vision is so frequently disturbed with migraine you could be in danger; and 5) if the attack is mild, carry on with what you're doing, if you feel safe to do so.

If you find you're starting an attack on waking—stay in bed and take your medication.

In any bad attack, 1) darken the room (you should have a room that has lined curtains for this purpose); 2) go to bed or lie down; and 3) apply a warm hot water bottle to the affected side of the head (some people find ice packs are better—you'll have to experiment).

Getting away from everything to rest is the best treatment. Ninety per cent of people with classical migraine improve within two hours if they lie down in a quiet, darkened room.

Miscarriage

A miscarriage is the loss of a foetus from the womb before the 28th week of pregnancy. After this time, if the baby is born dead it is called a stillbirth. Miscarriages most commonly occur up to the third month of pregnancy.

The problem very often is that a woman might not know whether she's actually miscarrying or whether she is simply having a late period. If the amount of bleeding is about what you would expect in a normal period—don't worry. **BUT** if the bleeding is heavier or goes on for more than two days, you'll need medical advice.

If you think you're miscarrying, don't use tampons even if you usually do; use sanitary towels and save them for your doctor to see. Go to bed and get someone to call for the doctor.

Should you have any uterine pains (like period pains or early labour pains when you're pregnant), go to bed and call the doctor even if at that stage there has been very little bleeding.

Motion sickness

Nausea and even vomiting are fairly common when travelling in any transport that rolls about. Planes and ships seem to be the worst offenders but many people are travel sick in cars or even trains. Anxiety is known to make matters worse and confidence is the best cure. This is less true of sea sickness than of the other kinds because here the abnormalities of motion can be very gross. Women are most severely affected, especially before their periods, and people with high blood pressure, sinusitis and migraine are also particularly susceptible.

There are several preventive measures that are worth trying: 1) don't read; 2) don't twist your neck; 3) place yourself so that you can see the moving horizon; 4) get fresh air; 5) avoid large and especially fatty meals before travelling on transport that makes you feel sick; and 6) take proprietary motion sickness tablets in the recommended dose but **NOT** if you're driving. If these don't work, see your doctor.

Should you ever have to travel by ambulance as company for someone else, keep facing forward and keep your eye on something outside. If you keep staring down at little Cathy's face you'll end up arriving at hospital feeling ill yourself.

Muscle cramps

Most cramps come on for no apparent reason and often occur in bed, though they may also occur after sudden chilling as in swimming. Loss of body salt from vomiting, sweating and prolonged diarrhoea can also cause cramps.

Cramps are easily overcome—especially if you have someone else handy to help. Simply stretch the muscle in cramp as strongly as you can. Cramps in the calf muscles can be cured by straightening the knee and pushing the sole of the foot upwards at the ankle. Cramps in the thigh are cured by pulling the leg well forward and straightening the knee and cramped fingers by pressing them out straight. For cramps in the foot—stand on the ball of the foot.

All of these procedures are even more effective if the cramped muscles are also massaged or warmed while being stretched.

Muscle strains

These are usually caused by overstretching a muscle or group of muscles and sometimes a part of the muscle may actually be torn. The strained areas are painful, may be swollen, bruised and make movement difficult.

Rest is the best cure and cold applications limit swelling and reduce pain. An elastic bandage can also be helpful. Apply it stretched under tension so that it gives support as you put on each turn. Overlap each turn so that no flesh gapes through between turns. Ask the person if it seems too tight. If he says it does, undo it all and start again. Do this too if the part beyond the bandage goes white or blue or causes the person any discomfort. Never use an elastic bandage around the knee, ankle, elbow or wrist without first covering the area with a large pad of cotton wool. This prevents damage to blood vessels and veins which lie close to the surface in these areas. Don't try to disperse the injury with exercises or heat lamps in the early stages as they may make matters worse.

N

Nervous breakdown 18, 30, 43, 44

It's very difficult to define what a nervous breakdown is and, strange though it may seem, it's a diagnosis that can often be made by the people surrounding the person rather than by the person himself or his doctor! Many people whose nerves are 'cracking up' have very good and rational explanations for their deterioration but their families and friends often seek help because **their** lives are becoming impossible. Nervous breakdowns don't usually happen dramatically although the onset may well be triggered off by bereavement, redundancy, divorce or the accumulation of many smaller stresses of everyday life.

People having nervous breakdowns start off by realising that they're not coping well with life and at this stage they blame themselves. Later the person loses control of the situation and becomes angry or despairing. The last stage is surprisingly a period of calmness. 'They'll have to do something now—I'm a dead loss' etc. So the stages are stress and pressure, loss of control, breaking point, letting go, anger and, finally, resignation.

Clearly, the best treatment is prevention. If anyone you know is going through any of these stages, seems to be worrying excessively, can't cope with work, doesn't want to get up in the mornings or sits around all day, you must encourage him to seek medical help. Don't wait until the whole thing blows up into a crisis. Should a crisis occur, try asking for the help of your family doctor first. If you have no luck, phone the *emergency Social Services Department* (look under Social Services in the front of your phone book). If the person is close to you, try to work out what the underlying cause might be. Many people get into this situation because of marital difficulties. You can go to a probation officer (look under Probation in the phone book) for help even if you are not on probation nor have ever had any contact with the courts. Your local Marriage Guidance counsellor may also be very helpful. All these people are helpful and used to dealing with crises such as these. Lastly, you could contact a local MIND group—there are 160 in the UK, so there is bound to be one near you.

Nettlerash (Urticaria or hives)

This extremely itchy, red, raised, blotchy rash is caused by a sensitivity to one of many different things. Its name arises because nettle stings produce the classical picture but other plants, jellyfish, insect bites or stings, certain foods (especially nuts, shellfish, pork, strawberries, onions and milk) and some drugs (especially aspirin and penicillin) can all cause it.

Treatment consists of removing the cause if you know what it is and in the meantime soothing the affected areas with calamine or other neutral, cool fluids. If you have some antihistamine tablets, take one even before seeing your doctor but don't use antihistamine cream as this can itself cause sensitivity in some people. Antihistamines can make you drowsy, so be careful if driving or operating machinery. Also don't take them with other drugs without checking with your doctor.

P

Painful periods (dysmenorrhoea)

Periods can and do hurt in many women and when added to pre-menstrual symptoms can make a woman's life (and that of her family) extremely unpleasant around period time.

Painful periods can be treated today with various hormones and which ones are used depends upon your type of period pain.

While your doctor is sorting out your hormone balance there are some useful first aid measures that can relieve the pain.

Hot baths help a lot, as do full doses of common painkillers. Some women may need to get a stronger painkiller from their doctor for the very worst days but otherwise it's best to use only aspirin or paracetamol in the recommended dose. A hot water bottle held over the lower tummy or between the legs also helps.

Many women say that they're more comfortable if they don't use tampons during the painful part of a period and it seems that being constipated makes matters worse too. If you regularly get pains that come to a head a couple of days **before** a period, you may have a condition called endometriosis, so see your doctor about treatment.

A little brandy or rum can produce excellent results but other food and drink should only be taken if you feel like it. Don't let anyone press food on you because it'll probably make you feel sick or even actually vomit. A good sleep is often helpful in relieving the pain.

Palpitation 14

A state in which one is conscious of one's heart beating rapidly. Palpitation is not usually a sign of heart disease and in young people is almost never so. As a generalisation, palpitation that arises abruptly and goes just as suddenly is more likely to be caused by heart disease than that which comes and goes slowly. If you have this first kind of palpitation or if you notice that your heart races in an irregular way—see your doctor.

Although palpitation can be very distressing, it is usually not dangerous (unless you know that you have high blood pressure or heart disease). The common type often responds to trick manoeuvres that stimulate the vagus nerve. Try tickling the back of the throat or pressing firmly over one eyeball. If neither of these works, lie down and rest. There is no rule of thumb as to how long attacks last or how frequently they occur. If you get them frequently or if they incapacitate you, see your doctor.

Simple preventive measures can help. Try 1) worrying less; 2) eating smaller meals, especially in the evening; 3) reducing your fatty food intake; 4) cutting out all tea and coffee; 5) asking your doctor's advice if you're on any pills as they may be causing the trouble; 6) cutting down or stopping smoking; and 7) cutting down or stopping drinking alcohol. Eventually you'll be able to re-introduce many of these items as you find out which are responsible.

Penis discharge

Almost always caused by venereal disease. See your local VD clinic or doctor as soon as you can. (See also page 110). Having said this though, this isn't in any way an emergency and should you first notice a discharge on a Saturday, it can wait until Monday for treatment. Nothing serious will happen in the meantime. **Don't** take any antibiotics you may have at home in an attempt to 'clear it up'. **Don't** ignore it; keep off alcohol (it makes it more painful to pass water); and keep off sex.

Make a note of your sex partners so that the doctor can contact them for treatment too. **Don't** delay seeking treatment hoping the discharge will go away. Getting VD isn't like catching a cold—it's serious and getting more difficult to treat unless it's caught early. Don't worry about having to give your identity, all clinics have a 'confidential' system.

Pregnancy 10, 22, 33, 35, 42

The way in which you view the idea that you might be pregnant depends very much on whether you planned the baby or not. If you are unmarried and don't really want to be pregnant or even if you're married and have an unplanned pregnancy, finding you **are** pregnant can be very bad news indeed. Obviously, if the baby is a wanted one, finding you're pregnant isn't any sort of emergency and you won't need to read on. But if you're pregnant and you don't want to be, **the main thing to do is to keep calm and not to panic.** There's no way that you can be **sure** you're not pregnant until six weeks and a day after the start of your last period because this is the first time that a pregnancy test can be relied on. In the meantime there's nothing anyone can do to tell definitely if you're pregnant. During this time a period may well appear and put your mind at rest anyway, so don't panic unnecessarily.

If you have a sympathetic general practitioner to whom you can talk, go and see him and tell him you think you're pregnant. He'll arrange for a pregnancy test. Take a specimen of urine passed as soon as you get up in the morning into a perfectly clean container. Should the result come back 'positive', then your doctor will refer you to a specialist at the local hospital to discuss having an abortion—if that is what you want.

Many people, however, don't feel able to discuss an abortion with their general practitioner for all kinds of reasons. If you feel this way, remember that you can go to the family planning clinic you have been attending and they will do a pregnancy test and advise you from there on.

There are two charitable organisations that can be of help too. *The British Pregnancy Advisory Service* (10) and the *Pregnancy Advisory Service* (42) are used to dealing with people in exactly this situation and can be relied upon for discretion. It is not widely known that on occasions these charities will be able to arrange for you to have an abortion under the NHS and so avoid paying their fees. They may also be able to make other arrangements if you cannot afford to pay.

The important thing to remember about having an abortion is that each day you delay after 12 weeks makes it more difficult for the doctor and more dangerous for you.

However worried you might feel, **DON'T** 1) drink gin to abort the baby—it simply won't work; 2) try getting rid of the pregnancy by taking a hot bath—this is no good either; 3) douche—it's a waste of time; 4) accept help from a friend; or 5) poke anything into your vagina.

There's no need to get desperate today. Wait until you know you're definitely pregnant and then take the action outlined above. If you do decide to go ahead with the pregnancy you will find *Gingerbread* (23) helpful.

R

Rupture

If you think you have ruptured yourself, don't panic—the chances of anything dramatic happening quickly are very slender. Usually there will be a swelling in the groin made larger by coughing or straining. Simply lie down with your knees bent and your head and shoulders supported by a pillow or two and get medical help. **Don't try pushing the swelling back in.** Operation is the treatment of choice, unless you are very old or ill, and results are excellent.

S

Scabies

This skin condition, also know as 'the itch', is caused by tiny mites which burrow under the skin and are just about visible to the naked eye. Scabies is slightly contagious, especially after close contact and produces severe itching. Scratching the skin can lead to secondary infection by bacteria.

The itching can be so intolerable that it keeps the sufferer awake at nights. You'll know it's scabies because there'll be a rash in one or more of these areas: 1) armpits; 2) waist; 3) between the thighs; 4) wrists; 5) between the knuckles.

Many people try to cure themselves with patent medicines and while some of these work, it's better to go to your doctor, who can arrange a complete and safe cure.

Sciatica 6

Not really a disease in its own right at all. Sciatica simply describes a pain, usually starting in the buttock and lower spine and running down the back of the leg to the calf. Raising the leg makes the pain worse and lying flat improves things.

Any pain like this needs full medical investigation, so don't delay. In the meantime, sleep on the floor or put a door or a thick plank under your mattress and use few pillows. Take ordinary painkillers until you get other stronger ones from your doctor. You'll find it helps to stay lying down even to eat and that a hot water bottle over the lower back or buttock helps enormously. Gentle massage can give relief and the pain usually goes within 3 weeks. If you suffer from this sort of back trouble, make sure that you have support in the small of the back when sitting in easy chairs or a car seat. Sit up—don't slump—it helps your spine.

Senile dementia 1, 30, 43

There are 7.1 million men and women over the age of 65 in the country today and this number is increasing, thanks to modern medical care. Unfortunately, this growth not only brings advantages but also disadvantages, one of which is the increasing number of old people who are deteriorating mentally as well as physically. About 1 person in 10 aged over 65 is thought to be demented.

Dementia is difficult to define but is a diffuse, non-specific deterioration of mental faculties which leads to an inability to cope with everyday living. Over the age of 80, a fifth of old people are thought to be in this state, so it's a serious problem. They are not 'mentally ill' of course, in the widely accepted sense of the word but simply can't cope safely with life without outside help. Memory loss is a real problem and sometimes produces life-threatening crises (such as leaving the stove on all night with its possible fire risk) which force relatives to seek help.

If you have an elderly relative or friend who's like this, get help early rather than late. *The Social Services Department* (look for the number in the front of the telephone directory under Social Services) will help and *Age Concern* are keen to help all they can. *MIND* will tell you how to contact a local group near you and between these three you should be able to sort something out. There may be an underlying medical condition that's causing the old person's problems but this isn't usually the case and these old folk don't need 'doctoring' as such.

Splinters

These are usually slivers of wood or thorns from bushes but splinters of glass and other materials can get stuck in the skin. You can remove a piece of glass that is nearly falling out but it's very easy to leave a fragment in a wound and you're better off going to a doctor who can make a more thorough search for deeply lodged pieces and then clean the wound. Never remove large glass splinters against resistance—you may do a lot of damage.

Splinters are important because they so often involve the hands and can go septic. They are especially painful and dangerous in the hands, not only because infection can soon render the hand so painful that it cannot be used but also because there are so many moving tendons (sinews) in the hand that can be damaged by infection. You don't need much to go wrong with your hands to make you realise how valuable they are.

The area around a simple small splinter should be washed gently, preferably with an antiseptic and then the projecting end of the splinter grasped between tweezers or cleaned fingernails.

If the splinter is not easily grasped, sterilize a sewing needle tip (by making it red hot in a flame), let it cool in the air and don't put it down anywhere, then **gently** tease the loose end of the splinter into a position in which you can remove it with tweezers. Never go digging deeply to remove the whole splinter or you might cause extra damage and get a serious infection of the tissues. If it looks as though the splinter is going to be difficult to remove, go to your doctor or local hospital.

A splinter under the nail is particularly painful and difficult to remove. Unless you can pull it out very easily, don't do anything else because you may break it whilst getting it out and so leave a piece deep under the nail which will be difficult even for a doctor to remove. When you get to hospital, the doctor can remove even quite deep splinters by making a V-shaped incision in the nail edge so as to allow him to get to the splinter. Only very rarely will all the nail have to come off. Never ignore splinters under nails—should they become infected, you may lose the nail and the infection might even damage the bone in the finger tip.

If any splinter draws blood, you should seek medical advice about an anti-tetanus injection.

Once you have removed a splinter, cover the area with a little antiseptic cream and apply an adhesive dressing until healed.

Strokes 14, 19, 46

A stroke is a sudden disturbance of brain function lasting for more than 24 hours caused by an interruption of the blood flow to the brain. Strokes are also called cerebro-vascular accidents (CVAs), cerebral thromboses, cerebral haemorrhages, apoplexy or shock. Strokes are usually caused by blood leaking into the brain from a burst artery or by an artery becoming blocked by a clot of blood.

The symptoms of a stroke range from a transitory disturbance of physical function and consciousness to deep unconsciousness and even death. When the person comes to, he's usually confused and can't think clearly. He may have a paralysis of his face, arm or leg on the whole of one side of his body with varying degrees of loss of sensation. His speech may also be altered. Some people wet themselves and others have visual disturbances. These signs may recover spontaneously in a few weeks or may be permanent. It all depends on how much damage was done in the brain when the stroke occurred.

Making the diagnosis of a stroke can be difficult at home but if you find someone unconscious with a floppy arm and/or leg on one side, you should suspect a stroke and call a doctor. The person may also have been incontinent from his bladder or bowel. While waiting for the doctor, keep the person as comfortable as possible and ensure that he can breathe properly (see page 20). If you have help, put him to bed gently.

Stye 21

A small boil or pustule on the edge of the eyelid usually starting in a hair follicle at the base of an eyelash.

Bathe the eye with cotton wool soaked in hot water and then throw the cotton wool away. Some people find cold tea on the cotton wool reduces the swelling and so makes a stye less painful.

Should the stye form a head, bathe the area gently with warm water, wash your hands and pluck out the eyelash at the base of the stye. This releases the pus and allows the stye to heal.

If you keep getting styes—see your doctor. If you work with food, keep away until your stye is healed.

Suicide 18, 27, 30, 43, 44, 48

There are two considerations here. 1) What to do if you find that someone has tried to kill himself. 2) What to do if you feel like killing yourself.

If you discover someone who you think has tried to kill himself, assess how ill he is. If you think he might be dead, turn to page 150. If he is still alive, carry out resuscitation procedures (see page 20 if he is not breathing and page 24 if there is no heart beat). Send for an ambulance at once or get someone else to do so while you try to revive him.

Should you ever feel like killing yourself, you can get help by calling your doctor. He will come if he possibly can. If you have no success, call the police or the Samaritans. The local Social Services Department also has a 24 hour emergency service—look under Social Services in the front of the telephone directory.

If you are desperate, don't stay alone. Talk to someone—this helps enormously. Either go to a friend, get him to come to you or talk to someone on the phone. The Samaritans are used to receiving just this sort of call and will help you over your immediate crisis. Once you're over this stage, see your doctor about it.

Anyone who threatens to take his own life must be helped by an expert but should someone tell you he's going to kill himself, don't panic. You may not need to get help at once but simply to talk to him quietly and reassuringly. Don't tell him 'not to be silly' and don't get angry. Stay calm, get over the immediate crisis and then get emergency help from the police, *Samaritans* (48) or Social Services Department. Many people threaten to kill themselves yet never do anything. Threats should always be taken seriously though and a watch kept for anyone stockpiling drugs of any kind that might be used in a future suicide attempt.

If you try to kill yourself, the chances are that you won't be compulsorily put into a mental hospital—at least, not the first time you try. Most people who try to kill themselves are not mentally ill in the commonly accepted sense of the phrase. They simply need help to overcome social or personal problems or perhaps need to be treated for a condition such as depression. It isn't illegal to try to kill yourself, so you won't get into trouble with the police. It is, of course, illegal to help someone else kill himself.

T

Teething

Teething babies can cause real havoc in any household because their sleep may be disturbed and this makes the parents lose sleep and become generally 'edgy'.

The best treatment for teething is to comfort your baby. If this doesn't work, soothing gels that you apply to the gums are helpful and can be used day and night. Teething powders are probably useless. Some children get relief by having something familiar to chew on.

Don't blame your baby's teething for all his ailments

If ever you're worried about your baby because he's ill, tell your doctor. Far too many mothers put things down to teething only to find their baby really has got something serious wrong which has been left to get worse.

Tetanus (Lockjaw)

This is a very dangerous infection caused by bacteria that live in soil entering the body through a break in the skin. Some people die from tetanus every year in the UK, so it's worth taking seriously. Although people imagine it is a disease exclusive to those working in agriculture, gardens and with horses, this is not true. Anyone can get lockjaw. In fact the group most 'at risk' are middle aged housewives, mainly because household dust can be just as dangerous as soil and because they often have not been protected by vaccination.

Any person who is badly wounded should have an anti-tetanus injection but many of the wounds that lead to tetanus go unnoticed in a day's gardening or housework or may be very tiny indeed.

The best way of avoiding tetanus is to make sure that you are immune by keeping your vaccine boosters up to date. All babies in this country get a course of tetanus immunisation as part of their triple vaccine course of three injections, each containing vaccine against diphtheria, whooping cough and tetanus. A booster needs to be given every five years or so after this to keep your immunity up and this can be done by your doctor or local hospital.

Should you think you've wounded yourself in a situation likely to cause tetanus and you're unprotected, don't panic—nothing will happen whilst going to the hospital where they will give a special new protective injection and an antibiotic to kill off the bacteria. They will also treat the wound of course.

Two commonly held misconceptions are 1) that you can **only** get tetanus by cutting yourself in the web between the thumb and forefinger, and 2) that tetanus is somehow caused by getting rust into a wound.

Toothache

This can vary in intensity from a mild pain lasting only a few seconds to a pain bad enough to keep you awake at night. The only way to deal with any kind of toothache is to go to a dentist for help.

In the meantime, take two aspirin or paracetamol tablets. **Never** place aspirin tablets against the gum beside an aching tooth as this can cause an unpleasant burn. Don't take any alcohol as this will make the toothache throb even more.

If there is swelling or soreness of the gums over a wisdom tooth, wash out your mouth with warm saline made by adding one teaspoon of salt to half a glass of warm water.

Oil of cloves is the old remedy for toothache but is only any good if the pain is caused by a large cavity or lost filling. In these cases a small piece of cotton wool soaked in oil of cloves can provide temporary relief until you see the dentist.

If you or your child falls over and breaks a tooth it can be rendered less painful while waiting to get to a dentist by bathing the broken edge in alcohol (whiskey will do). This kills the surface cells and so makes the broken edge less sensitive.

If a child knocks a permanent tooth out or loosens it badly, go to a dentist or accident department without delay as often there is hope of the tooth taking when placed back in the socket and this is important cosmetically.

U

Urine retention

The inability to pass water. Most commonly seen in elderly men with an enlarged prostate gland that presses on the outlet from the bladder. Also seen in children with a tight foreskin and women with fibroids, a displaced womb or gonorrhoea.

Sit in a warm bath to pass water or try passing water with a hot water bottle on your abdomen. Call the doctor or go to your local casualty department if you can get there.

The underlying cause always needs treatment, so don't put off getting medical help.

V

Vaginal discharge

All women experience a vaginal discharge at some time during their lives, even if it's only the normal discharge that occurs around the middle of the menstrual cycle, at ovulation, during pregnancy or whilst on the Pill.

But these do not compare with the excruciatingly itchy irritation of an acute attack of vaginal thrush. This usually comes about because the vaginal area is kept too warm and moist by wearing trousers, tights or nylon pants. Women who wear skirts, cotton pants and stockings are much less likely to get this infection. The monilia organism takes a hold in suitable warm, wet surroundings and seems mostly to affect women who are run down physically or mentally, pregnant, on the Pill or suffering from diabetes.

As soon as you see the white, curdy monilial discharge you should 1) make up a solution of one teaspoonful of vinegar or lemon juice in one pint of water, crouch over a bowl in the bath and splash the solution forcibly into your vagina; and 2) get out of the bath and dry yourself and then push a small amount of fresh, live yoghurt into your vagina. You could try coating a tampon in the yoghurt and then pushing it well up inside. The yoghurt contains organisms that will combat the yeasty monilia and can bring relief very quickly. If you use a contraceptive foam, use your applicator to get the yoghurt inside your vagina.

Don't wear a pad and don't wear tampons if you have this type of vaginal discharge. Wear disposable paper pants if you have them; boil your pants after use if you're wearing cotton ones; and preferably wear no pants at all. Wear stockings and a skirt instead.

All this is only by way of immediate self-help and is no substitute for seeing your doctor. He can give you pessaries, creams or tablets to cure the condition completely and will be able to see if there is any underlying cause for your having got it in the first place.

VD

Venereal diseases are by definition conditions that are caught by sexual intercourse. Unfortunately VD is a complex group of conditions and because so many people (especially women) simply carry the disease yet are unaffected as far as they are aware, this means it can be spread very easily.

You should go to a VD clinic (or your doctor) if you or your partner has any of the following: 1) itching, soreness or discharge from the vagina, penis or anus; 2) a sore lump or rash in the genital area, around the anus or in the mouth; or 3) increased frequency of passing water or pain on doing so. If you have any of these, stop all sexual activity and get help as soon as possible.

You can go straight to a special clinic and no introductory letter is needed. These clinics are geared to diagnose and treat any

disease that is sexually transmitted and can refer you elsewhere if you don't have VD. To find out where special clinics are, 1) look for posters in public lavatories, health centres or post offices; 2) look in the telephone directory under Veneral Disease. (Some areas even have recorded telephone messages that give you information about where to go); or 3) phone or visit your local hospital casualty department and ask for information.

At the special clinic you'll be given a number and all your records will be confidential. The doctor will want to know 1) the symptoms you've had; 2) what sex partners you've had in the last three months and whether you could contact them again; 3) if you're allergic to drugs; and 4) if you've had anal or oral contact. Homosexual sex can transmit VD too, so don't be offended if the doctor asks you about this.

If caught early enough, most VD can be easily treated. Don't delay.

Vomiting

This is mainly caused by conditions inside the abdomen or, less commonly, by conditions related to the brain. Gastritis or gastroenteritis are by far the commonest cause of vomiting but pregnancy vomiting (which need not be confined to the early morning) is also fairly common. In children, the commonest cause of vomiting is tonsillitis and don't forget that whooping cough may present as vomiting too. Certain conditions in the head can also cause vomiting, including migraine, Ménière's disease, travel sickness, vertigo and meningitis.

It is difficult to give a rule of thumb about vomiting because it affects people in such different ways and may or may not be a sign of a serious underlying condition. It's fair to say though that if you vomit for longer than either the daylight or nighttime hours—you need medical help. Children and young babies especially can become dangerously ill if they vomit a lot so if your child or baby vomits for more than six hours, tell your doctor.

It's wise to call a doctor: 1) if you vomit any black or bloody material; 2) if you have a stiff neck; 3) if you are dizzy when you vomit; or 4) if you have a sudden onset of abdominal pain.

If ever your child vomits so forcibly that the vomit is thrown a very long way, tell your doctor.

When it comes to treatment, there is little to be done. Treat the cause if you can and in the meantime lie flat and take nothing by mouth until a couple of hours have passed. Sips of iced water are good and small amounts of milk may settle the stomach. Plain water in large amounts tends to induce further vomiting. As soon as you feel better and can keep drinks down, drink plenty of fruit juices, well diluted—it's amazing how much fluid you lose by vomiting and this very dehydration makes you feel worse than you need be.

you can do to treat worms yourself, so get medical help. There is certainly no need to feel guilty as the cleanest, best cared for children can get worms.

In the meantime take care to flush away any wormy stools and wash out potties with disinfectant. Take particular care with lavatory seat cleanliness and boil nappies or pants separately from your other washing. Keep your child's nails clean and short, wash his hands and yours after helping him in the lavatory and, if necessary, give him cotton gloves to prevent him from scratching at night. Change the child's sheets daily and hoover around his bed to remove worm eggs carried in dust.

Don't be alarmed if the doctor suggests treating the other children and even the adults in the family—it's better to be safe and the treatment is simple and harmless. Don't attempt any home treatment. 'Wormcakes' are useless.

W

Worms

These can be very upsetting to both parent and child. Firstly, many parents feel it is shameful or 'dirty' that their child should have worms and, secondly, the child is distressed by the irritation. There is nothing

1 Age Concern England,
Bernard Sunley House,
60 Pitcairn Road,
Mitcham,
Surrey CR4 3LL
01 640 5431

2 AL-ANON (for relatives of
problem drinkers),
61 Great Dover Street,
London SE1 4YF
01 403 0888

3 Alcoholics Anonymous,
140a Tachbrook Street,
London SW1V 2NE
01 834 8202

4 Association for Improvements in
the Maternity Services, (AIMS)
Secretary: Ms Christine Rogers,
163 Liverpool Road,
London N1 0RS
01 278 5628

5 Asthma Society and Friends of the
Asthma Research Council,
St Thomas's Hospital,
Lambeth Palace Road,
London SE1 7EH
01 261 0110

6 Back Pain Association,
31–33 Park Road,
Teddington,
Middlesex TW11 0AB
01 977 5474

7 British Diabetic Association,
10 Queen Anne Street,
London W1M 0BD
01 323 1531

8 British Epilepsy Association,
Crowthorne House,
Bigshotte,
New Wokingham Road,
Wokingham,
Berks RG11 3AY
0344 773122

9 British Migraine Association,
178A High Road,
Byfleet,
Weybridge,
Surrey KT14 7ED
91 52468

10 British Pregnancy Advisory
Service,
Austy Manor,
Wootton,
Wawen,
Solihull,
West Midlands B95 6BX
05642 3225

11 British Red Cross Society,
National Headquarters,
9 Grosvenor Crescent,
London SW1X 7EJ
01 235 5454.
For County Branches
see local directories.

12 British Rheumatism and Arthritis
Association,
6 Grosvenor Crescent,
London SW1X 7ER
01 235 0902

13 Cancer Research Campaign,
Secretary: Mr T. A. Moore,
Ailsa,
86 Sywell Road,
Overstone,
Northampton NN6 0AQ
0604 43860

14 The Chest, Heart and Stroke
Association,
Tavistock House North,
Tavistock Square,
London WC1H 9JE
01 387 3012/7291

15 The Compassionate Friends,
National Secretary:
Mrs Gill Hodder,
5 Lower Clifton Hill,
Clifton,
Bristol BS8 1BT
0272 292 778

16 Cruse,
Cruse House,
126 Sheen Road,
Richmond,
Surrey TW9 1UR
01 940 4818

17 Depressives Anonymous,
Hon. Secretary: Ms Pat Freya,
83 Derby Road,
Nottingham NG1 5BB

18 Disabled Drivers' Association,
Registered Office,
Ashwellthorpe Hall,
Ashwellthorpe,
Norwich NR16 1EX
050 841 449

19 Disabled Living Foundation,
346 Kensington High Street,
London W14 8NS
01 602 2491

20 Family Planning Association,
Margaret Pyke House,
27–35 Mortimer Street,
London W1N 7RJ
01 636 7866

21 Gingerbread,
35 Wellington Street,
London WC2E 7BN
01 240 0953

22 La Leche League,
P.O. Box 3424,
London WC1N 3XX
01 404 5011

23 Mastectomy Association,
26 Harrison Street,
King's Cross,
London WC1

24 Mental Patients Union,
Secretary: Mr Ken Wood,
137 Lavender Hill,
Battersea,
London SW11
01 223 2580

25 Migraine Trust,
45 Great Ormond Street,
London WC1N 3HD
01 278 2676

26 National Association for the Divorced and Separated, Secretary: Ms Margaret A. Newey, 13 High Street, Little Shelford, Cambridge CB2 5ES Watford 22181

27 National Association for Mental Health (MIND). 22 Harley Street, London W1N 2ED 01 637 0741

28 National Association for Maternal and Child Welfare, 1 South Audley St, London W1Y 6JS 01 491 1315

29 National Association for the Welfare of Children in Hospital, Argyle House, 29–31 Euston Road, London NW1 2SD

30 National Childbirth Trust, 9 Queensborough Terrace, London W2 3TB 01 221 3833

31 National Council on Alcoholism, 3 Grosvenor Crescent, London SW1X 7EE 01 235 4182

32 National Council for One Parent Families, 255 Kentish Town Road, London NW5 2LX 01 267 1361

33 National Council for Voluntary Organisations, 26 Bedford Square, London WC1 01 636 4066

34 National Institute of Adult Continuing Education, 19B De Montfort Street, Leicester LE1 7GE 0533 551451

35 National Schizophrenia Fellowship, 78/79 Victoria Road, Surbiton, Surrey KT6 4NS 01 390 3651/2/3

36 National Society for the Prevention of Cruelty to Children, 67 Saffron Hill, London EC1 01 580 8812

37 Parents Anonymous Croydon and Tandridge: in local phone book or press, or phone 01 668 4805 (24 hour service) for details of local groups.

38 Patients Association, Room 33, 18 Charing Cross Road, London WC2H 0HR 01 240 0671

39 Pregnancy Advisory Service, 11–13 Charlotte Street, London W1P 1HD 01 637 8962

40 Relatives of the Mentally Ill, Langer Weg 6, 7300 Esslingen, Germany.

41 RoSPA, Cannon House, The Priory Queensway, Birmingham B4 6BS 021 233 2461

42 The Royal Association for Disability and Rehabilitation (incorporating The British Council for Rehabilitation of the Disabled and The Central Council for the Disabled) 25 Mortimer Street, London W1N 8AB 01 637 5400

43 Safety in Playgrounds Action Group, 16 Old Hall Road, Salford, Manchester M7 0JH

44 The Samaritans, 17 Uxbridge Road, Slough SL1 1SN In local phone book or press.

45 Schizophrenia Association of Great Britain, Hon Secretary: Mrs Hemmings, BSc, Tyr Twr, Llanfair Hall, Caenarvon LL55 1TT 0248 670 379

46 The National Federation of Solo Clubs, 7–8 Ruskin Chambers, 191 Corporation Street, Birmingham 4 021 236 2879

47 Spinal Injuries Association, General Secretary: Ms Tyrrell, 5 Crowndale Road, London NW1 1TU 01 388 6849/0

48 The Sports Council, 16 Upper Woburn Place, London WC1H 0QP 01 388 1277

49 Cystitis sufferers Angela Kilmartin, 75 Mortimer Road, London N1 5AR

50 Women's National Cancer Control Campaign, 1 South Audley Street, London W1Y 5DQ 01 499 7532/3/4

We are fortunate in the UK in not having many biting and stinging animals and insects. Bees and wasps sting, a few insects bite and only one type of snake is dangerous—the adder.

Most people suffer only temporary discomfort from the majority of stings and bites but real emergencies can occur when:

1 The sting involves the mouth or throat.

2 The person's body over-reacts to the injected poison and instead of suffering mild pain and irritation, he becomes very distressed and may even have breathing difficulties.

In either case—**get medical help at once**. In the second case, treat for shock while awaiting help (See page 34).

Bee stings:

A bee leaves its sting in the flesh but it can easily be removed with tweezers or clean finger nails. You can also 'wipe' it out with a pin or needle held flat to the skin. Be careful when removing the sting not to squeeze the poison sac. If you grip the sting very low down near the skin you should have no trouble. Apply a cold dressing or calamine lotion or hold the area under cold water.

Wasp stings:

These leave no barb in the skin. Place some lemon juice or vinegar on the sting. If you accidentally eat a wasp as it sits on food the sting can be dangerous. Take cold drinks; eat ice cubes and get medical help.

Bee

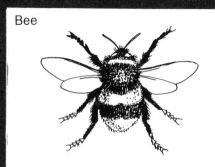

Bee sting

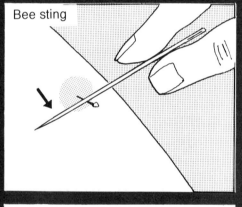

Wasp

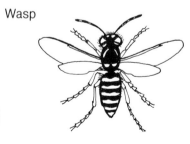

Insect stings:
Horseflies, mosquitoes, gnats, fleas, bedbugs and sandflies are all possible causes of insect stings in the UK. None produces a problem except in highly susceptible people who should be treated for shock. (See page 34). Soothing lotions are helpful and antihistamine tablets give relief if the person has been bitten in many places. Surgical spirit is also soothing. (See also scabies, page 104).

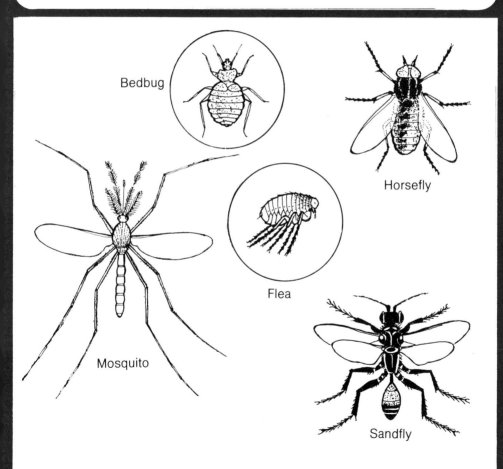

Bedbug

Horsefly

Flea

Mosquito

Sandfly

Snake bites:

In the UK there are only 3 main types of snake and only one is venomous.

The adder **(a)** usually lives in clearings or on the edge of woodlands, on moors, hills, railway cuttings and mountains. It is grey, yellow or reddish brown, about 75cm (30″) long and has a broad head. The main features are the black zig-zag markings on its back. The harmless, smooth snake and grass snake have spots on their backs. Adder bites are painful and may produce sweating, vomiting and diarrhoea, stomach pains and even loss of consciousness. They rarely cause death. Adders only bite a person in self-defence and inject only a little venom.

Action:

1 Rest the person.
2 Immobilise the bitten part.
3 Reassure the person that he won't die.
4 Give painkilling tablets.
5 Get him to hospital quickly.

Don't

1 Suck the venom out.
2 Apply a tourniquet.
3 Cut the bite.
4 Put any chemicals on.

Animal bites and scratches:

Scratches from domestic animals are rarely troublesome.

1 Clean the area with disinfectant. Put a light, dry dressing on.
2 Deep scratches should be seen by a doctor.
3 All animal bites need medical attention because the deep punctures of animal teeth carry infection (possibly including tetanus in the UK and rabies in some parts of the world) deep into the tissues.

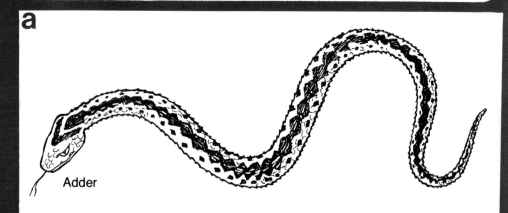

a

Adder

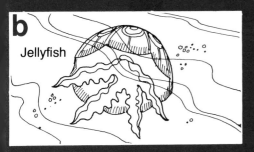

b Jellyfish

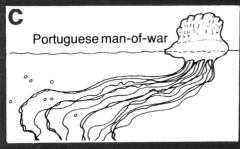

c Portuguese man-of-war

Jellyfish stings:

If jellyfish (**b**) are around, keep a look out and don't swim near them.

If you are stung, get to the shore, cover your hands with sand and then pick off any adherent pieces of jellyfish.

Apply a soothing cream or lotion. Should you be stung by a jellyfish it's probably wise to get medical help because there is one poisonous (though not lethal) type—the Portuguese man-of-war—for which medical treatment may be necessary (**c**). This jellyfish can be identified by the 'sail' it puts up in the form of an inflated bladder.

Don't forget that the stinging tentacles float 'downstream' in the current, so keep away from the back of the jelly mass. (The tentacles can be up to 45m (50 yards) long).

Plant stings:

Nettles (**d**) and a few other plants in the UK do sting but they are harmless and the stings are usually easily treated with soothing lotions. A dock leaf rubbed on works wonders too.

If you get anything other than simple itching and pain, see a doctor.

Some plants, especially those of the primula family, do not actually sting but produce severe skin reactions in those susceptible people who come into contact with them. The dermatitis so caused can be very unpleasant and may need medical treatment. Obviously people who are sensitive in this way should be careful never to come into contact with the plant again.

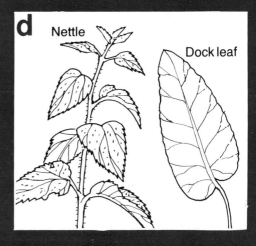

d Nettle   Dock leaf

Eyes

1 Never try to remove anything embedded in or stuck to the surface of the eye—leave this to a doctor.
2 Never touch any foreign body that is lodged on the coloured part of the eye—get medical help.
3 If ever in doubt about a damaged eye, cover it up and get medical help.

Getting rid of an object in the eye:

1 Get the person to blink repeatedly—the increased tear flow plus the blinking may wash the object out. Blowing the nose also helps.
2 If the object can be seen loose or can be felt by the person to be under the upper or lower lid:
i Wash your hands.

iia Take a piece of cotton wool or a freshly laundered handkerchief and twist a corner so as to produce a firm point.
iii Sit the person down in a good light. Stand behind him and pull down the lower lid to see if the object is there. If it is, dislodge it with the pointed cotton wool or handkerchief held in your other hand.
3 Most foreign bodies stick under the upper lid. Pulling the upper lid down over the lower lid can sometimes dislodge the object but the best thing to do is to:
Lay a match over the upper lid, **(b)**, parallel to the edge; hold it firmly in place with a finger of one hand and press gently down as you lift the lid

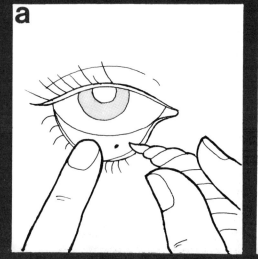

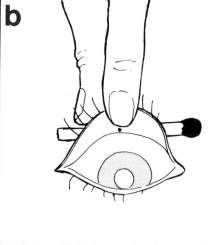

edge up by the lashes with the other hand. You bend the lid back over the match as if the match were a hinge. This will reveal the under side of the lid and hopefully the foreign body.

4 If there is any danger to the surface of the eye, get medical help.

5 Never use a sharp instrument or tweezers to remove anything from the eye.

6c Any corrosive fluid (or indeed any fluid other than water) splashed into the eye must be washed out **at once:** Get the person to hold his face under water in a basin and then to open and close his eyes. If he can't do this, put his eye under a **gently running** tap for a few minutes. If he can't do this, pour water from a cup or jug on to the eye.

Ears

The commonest problem with ears is in children who stick things in them. Beads, matches and small toys are most often found.

After a fall (with or without loss of consciousness) a person may lose blood and/or straw-coloured fluid from the ear. If ever you see this, get medical help at once—the person may have fractured his skull.

Objects in the ears

1 Never poke the ear yourself as you may damage the delicate ear drum.

2 Try leaning the child over to the affected side and then gently dislodge the object if it is only just inside.

3 If this produces no result, go to a doctor.

Noses

Again the most common problem at home is the child who sticks a bead, bean or toy up his nose.

1 Get the child to blow out through his nose while you shut off the other nostril. This sometimes dislodges the object.

2 Never try to remove anything unless it is easily held with tweezers and lies very superficially. Never poke about deep in the nose.

Just as with ears, should anyone ever have a nose bleed or the loss of pale fluid from the nose after a fall or head injury, get medical help to come at once.

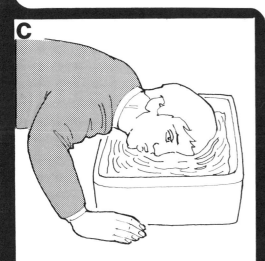 C

For nose bleeds see page 32.

Disease	Most often seen in	Site of rash	Type of rash
Chicken pox.	Children.	Mostly head and body. Arms and legs spared.	Crops of red spots blister and form scabs which drop off after 10 days.
German measles.	Older children.	Behind ears, forehead. Spreads to rest of body.	Flat, pink spots which may merge to cover body with pink flush.
Urticaria (hives, nettlerash).	Anybody, especially allergic people.	Variable, according to cause.	Raised wheals which may be surrounded by reddened skin and may appear in crops.
Insect bites and stings.	Anybody.	Variable.	A sensitised person may develop urticaria.
Measles.	Children under 6.	Neck, face, trunk, arms, and legs.	Small, red, flat or raised spots may merge and completely cover skin in severe cases.

...en rash appears	Other signs	Action
–21 days after contact.	Fever, itching.	Relieve itching with calamine lotion. Cut nails to reduce damage from scratching. Child infectious from 24 hours before spots appear until they're all covered with scabs.
◄–21 days after contact.	Swollen, tender glands behind ears and in back of neck.	Beware of contact with pregnant women as German measles can cause foetal abnormality. Child infectious from 7 days before rash appears until 4 days after.
...ay be due to allergy to food, ...ants, drugs, blood transfusion, ...sect bites or stings, infection ...nd, rarely, pollen.	May itch intensely.	Take antihistamine tablets if necessary. Soothe skin with calamine lotion.
...fter bites or stings, eg, wasps, ...ees, fleas, mosquitoes, lice ...nd horseflies.	Itching.	Soothing lotion on bite or sting. Take antihistamine tablets if necessary.
...4 days after contact.	Cough, cold, runny nose, pink eyes, fever, eyes painful in bright light, small, white spots on inside of cheeks.	Protect eyes from bright light. Call doctor if worried, especially if ears are painful. Child infectious from 7th day after exposure until 5 days after rash has gone.

Disease	Most often seen in	Site of rash	Type of rash
Pityriasis rosea.	Young adults.	Trunk, arms and legs.	Single, bright red 'he patch' followed by pinkish, oval, scaly patches a week later.
Prickly heat.	Anybody.	Where sweat glands are most numerous. In babies on cheeks, neck, trunk and nappy area.	Small, red spots or general pinkness of skin.
Roseola.	Children under 3.	Generalised.	Small, pink spots.
Scabies.	Anybody.	Armpits, waist, ankles, inside wrists, between fingers, palms, round nipples, penis.	Red spots, sometimes with blisters. May have urticaria. Scratch mark
Scarlet fever.	Children.	Starts on neck, groins and armpits and spreads to rest of body. Notably absent around mouth.	Tiny red, raised spots a flushed skin. Often becomes scaly as it heals.
Shingles.	Adults, especially the old.	Usually chest and abdomen but can affect face. Runs in bands, usually around one side of body.	Crops of red spots blister then scab.

en rash appears	Other signs	Action
	May be some itching, fever and headache.	Calamine lotion to reduce itching.
er overheating, especially if eat builds up	Hot, sweaty skin.	Remove some clothing and reduce room temperature. Wear cotton underwear, not wool. Avoid synthetic material for clothing. A cool bath or calamine lotion to soothe skin.
10 days after contact.	High fever suddenly falls after 3–4 days as short-lived rash appears.	None. A mild condition that is often not diagnosed.
er contact with scabies fferer.	Itching relatives or sex partner.	See doctor for treatment.
5 days.	Headache, loss of appetite, sore throat, vomiting and abdominal pain.	Get medical help because complications can occur.
er infection with virus robably the same as that of icken pox).	Fever. Pain and tenderness precede rash and may remain afterwards.	Calamine lotion to relieve itching. Pain killers. Get medical advice.

Soccer
1 Sprained ankles (see page 44)
2 Bruised shins
3 Muscle strains (see page 100)

Rugby
1 Damage to knee ligaments
2 Head injuries (see pages 43, 78)
3 Fractures (see page 36)

Athletics
1 Muscle strains (see page 100)
2 Achilles' tendon strain
3 Irritation of the knee cap

Cricket
1 Laceration from ball (see page 31)
2 Finger injuries and fractures (see page 39)
3 Hand dislocations (see page 44)

Squash
1 Laceration of head (see page 31)
2 Eye injuries
3 Muscle strains and pulls (see pages 100)

Gymnastics
1 Muscle sprains and strains (see pages 44, 100)
2 Wrist injuries
2 Back trouble

Hockey
1 Cuts from sticks (see pages 30–31)
2 Bruised shins
3 Bruising from ball

Swimming
1 Shoulder injuries
2 Lacerations (see page 31)
3 Inhalation of water (see page 142)

Badminton
1 Muscle strains (see page 100)
2 Sprains (see page 44)
3 Tennis elbow

Riding
1 Concussion (see pages 43, 78)
2 Fractures (see page 36)
3 Thigh muscle strains (see page 100)

Not breathing
|
Mouth to mouth
resuscitation (see pages
20–21)
|
Hospital

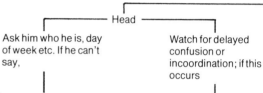

Head

Ask him who he is, day
of week etc. If he can't
say,
|
Hospital

Watch for delayed
confusion or
incoordination; if this
occurs
|
Hospital

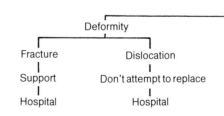

Deformity

Fracture
|
Support
|
Hospital

Dislocation
|
Don't attempt to replace
|
Hospital

ERSON

Breathing

Unconscious
|
Recovery position
(see page 79)
|
Check airway
|
Observe
|
Hospital

**Been unconscious
momentarily**
|
Observe off the pitch
|
No play for 10 days

Conscious

Injury

Neck
|
Do not move
|
Able to move limbs?
|
Tingling or burning in the
limbs?
|
Make a neck collar
(made by folding large
size newspaper three
times over and joining
with adhesive tape)
|
Hospital

Trunk
|
If sharp pain on
breathing or abdominal
pain lasting five minutes
|
Hospital

Limbs

Full movement without
weight on affected part

No
|
bone tenderness,
swelling, loss of power,
possible fracture
|
Hospital

Yes
|
Can he bear partial
weight?
|
Can he bear full weight?

If so, resume.

Laceration
|
Firm dressing
|
May need stretcher
|
May need tetanus
innoculation
|
Hospital

Tummy ache or abdominal pain can be caused by lots of different conditions ranging from eating too many green apples to cancer.

Deciding which is causing a particular abdominal pain can be very difficult even for a doctor but certain areas of the abdomen are more often affected by particular painful conditions which makes the position of the pain helpful to the doctor when making a diagnosis. The diagrams on the right should only be used as a rough guide for your own information. **It is no substitute for your doctor making a proper diagnosis.**

The problem is, when to get medical help. **In children,** be guided by how your child seems to you. If you're at all worried, especially about a baby—**get medical help at once.** Especially get help if a baby has vomiting or diarrhoea for more than six hours. Babies can lose fluid easily like this and very quickly go downhill. If in doubt with any child **always call your doctor.**

With adults, there's usually not such a need for urgency. Be guided by the following rules:

Get medical help for:

1 Any pain of sudden onset that is severe enough to make you want to lie down.
2 Any abdominal pain lasting more than 12 hours.
3 Any pain that makes you vomit for more than an hour or two.

4 Abdominal pain associated with vomiting blood; passing black or very dark stools; a recent loss of weight; yellowness of the skin or whites of the eyes; passing water frequently (especially if it is painful to do so).

Things the doctor will want to know:

1 How long you have had the pain.
2 Is it like anything you've had before?
3 Is it getting better or worse?
4 In which part of the tummy the pain first started.
5 What the pain is like (knife-like, throbbing, squeezing etc.)
6 Where it is worst now.
7 Where it goes to.
8 What brought it on.
9 What makes it better.
10 Date of last menstrual period.
11 Other related complaints.

If you can answer these questions the doctor will be able to sort out the problem more quickly.

By and large, abdominal pain alone (with no other trouble) isn't likely to be anything serious. **BUT** don't wait until the person is so ill that you have to call a doctor—always act sooner rather than later, especially at night or weekends. Too many people leave calling the doctor until they're desperate and then get upset and so add to their problems when they can't get him immediately.

Action

For immediate relief:

1 Go to bed.
2 Take only small sips of water by mouth if you want something to drink.
3 Place a covered hot water bottle on your tummy.
4 Get help if you feel worse.
5 Don't take pain killers—if the pain is that bad, get medical help.

Some common causes of longstanding abdominal pain.

Pain at 1—Hiatus hernia
(stomach hernia into chest).
Pain at 2—Gall bladder disease.
Pain at 3—Diverticular disease.
Pain at 4—Ulcers and other gastric
disorders. Stomach cancer.
NOTE. Any pain, however slight, that goes on for a week or more must be investigated by a doctor.

Some common causes of sudden onset abdominal pain

Pain at 1—Hiatus hernia.
Heartburn.
Gall bladder disease.
Pain at 2—Ulcers.
Gastritis.
Indigestion.
Inflammation of the
pancreas (pain may go
through to the back).
Pain at 3—Gall bladder disease.
Pain at 4—Appendicitis.
Pain at 5—Appendicitis.
Pain at 6—Inflammation of fallopian
tubes.
Pain at 7—Cystitis (bladder
inflammation).
Pain at 8—Diverticular disease.
Pain at 9—Loin pain (coming from back
and into groin). Kidney pain
(probably stones).

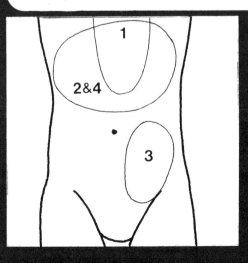
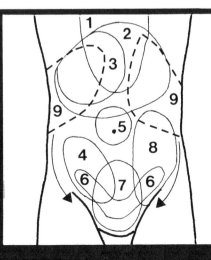

Fits

These can be frightening, especially the first time you see them.

Signs

1 The person falls down, usually without warning, loses consciousness and may make strange noises and cry out. He may froth at the mouth and may have some blood in his mouth where he's bitten his tongue. The person may also wet himself.

2 There will also be involuntary convulsive movements of the limbs.

3 Petit mal (minor) fits are often barely noticeable and show as a momentary blankness or loss of reality for a few seconds. In this type of fit the person rarely falls but carries on with his normal life.

Action

For major fits:

1 Keep calm and leave the person where he is unless he's actually damaging himself by hitting his limbs against nearby objects.

2 Remove furniture so that he doesn't damage himself further, or pull him gently away from hazards (fire, traffic etc).

3a Put something soft under his head and loosen his collar, tie and tight clothing.

4 When the attack is over, let him lie quietly or sleep and make sure that someone is with him in the period of confusion that often follows a fit. (See page 79 for recovery position).

Don't

1 Restrain convulsive movements forcibly: they're so strong that you may damage his muscles as they pull against your restraint. Light restraint to stop the patient damaging himself is all that is required.

Don't

2 Put anything in the mouth—this is now thought to be useless and anyway can be difficult to do. Bitten tongues heal—broken teeth never do.

Don't

3 Give anything to drink during the attack.

Don't

4 Call the doctor (for a brief uncomplicated attack) unless one attack follows another without the person regaining consciousness in between.

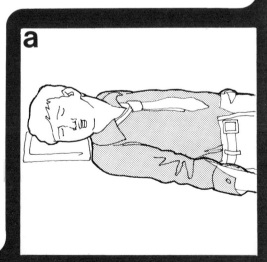
a

Fainting

A sudden loss of consciousness, usually precipitated by:

1 A stuffy, hot room.
2 An emotional shock.
3 Severe pain.
4 An unpleasant sight (road accident, injection needle etc). Unlike many other causes of unconsciousness, there is usually a warning. The person feels 'heady', sways, complains of giddiness, has a pale face and beads of cold sweat.

Action

1b Lie the person down and lift up the legs briefly to return blood to the head by gravity.
2 Loosen tight clothing.
3 Open windows to get air to him.
4 Turn him into the recovery position (see page 78).

5c Take the pulse—it will be slow: 40–50/minute, so confirming a faint.

Never give any drinks to an unconscious person. Once he has come round and is able to hold a cup himself unaided, he can have a drink.

If the person hasn't come round within a few minutes, get medical help as it might not be a faint.

It can sometimes be difficult to distinguish between a fit or a faint especially as some faints can be accompanied by jerking or incontinence of urine. The best way of telling which is which (and this can only be done in retrospect) is to ask if the person had any warning sensations. Faints are usually preceded by these sensations and fits may be followed by confusion, headache, or sleeping, which faints are not.

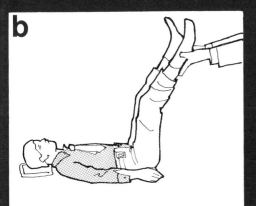

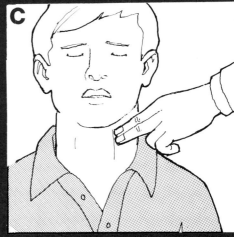

Things you'll need:
1 A bed with a pillow and blankets.
2 A waterproof sheet, polythene carrier bags broken open or newspaper to go under the sheet.
3 An ordinary sheet.
4 A table to put things on.
5 A large clean basin for hot water.
6 A large towel to wrap the baby in.
7 Soap and a clean towel for washing yourself and the mother.
8 Scissors and three 23cm (9in) lengths of string (boil both for 10 minutes in a saucepan and leave there until needed). Elastic bands (unboiled) will do if you have no string.
9 A cot for the baby.
10 A helper if possible.
11 Make all possible efforts to get a doctor or midwife but if you can't, don't panic—birth is a natural process and a woman will probably cope perfectly well if you are calm and reassure her, especially if she has had a baby before.

The First stage of labour (usually lasts several hours):

Signs may include:
1 Regular contractions in the lower abdomen.
2 Low backache.
3 A 'show' of bloodstained mucus from the birth canal.
4 A loss of fluid from the birth canal as the bag of water containing the baby breaks.

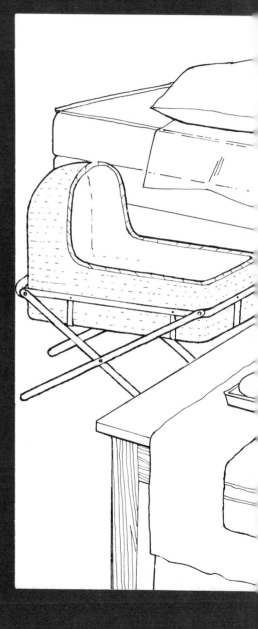

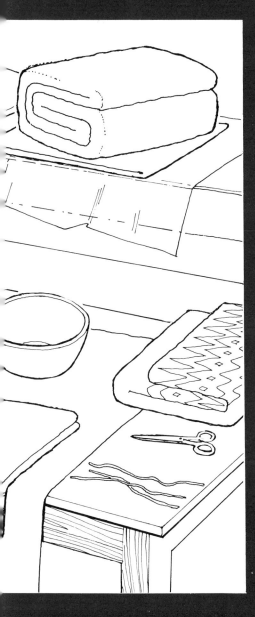

Action:
1 Let the woman do whatever she feels most comfortable doing. If her waters have broken she should not be upright until a midwife or doctor says that it is safe.
2 Get her to empty her bladder (in a chamber pot and not in the lavatory just in case the birth is sudden).
3a Reassure her and stay with her.

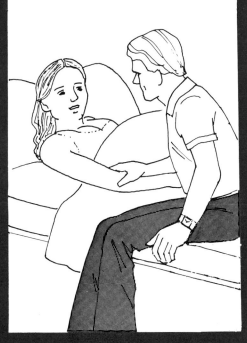

a

The Second Stage of Labour
(lasts hours or minutes, usually shorter after previous babies):

Signs: The woman feels a strong desire to push down.

Action:
1 Wash your hands and scrub your nails.
2 Encourage the woman to bear down **with** her contractions. She should not push in her pain-free intervals. Get her to relax then. Support the woman in whichever position she feels most comfortable.

The Birth

Signs: A bulge appears at the opening of the birth canal—this is usually the baby's head but can be its bottom.

Action:
1 Ask the woman to **stop pushing.**
2 Wash the area around the vaginal opening and wash away any bowel motions that might have appeared from the back passage.
3 Tell the woman to pant with her mouth open with each contraction.
4 As the baby emerges, control the head so that it doesn't 'pop' out. If necessary, push on it firmly so it comes out steadily.

5a Dont't interfere at all with the baby as it comes out unless the cord is around its neck. If so, unloop it quickly and gently. If there is a membrane across the baby's face, break it.

6b Support the head in your hands as the shoulders are born. This is the widest part and from now on the baby slips out easily.
7 Hook your fingers under his armpits, support the chest and when he's out, either lie him on the bed between the mother's thighs or put him on her tummy. Tell her what sex it is.

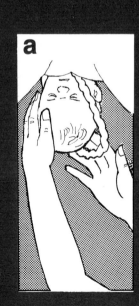

a

8 Wipe his mouth and eyes with a clean piece of cotton wool and make sure he's breathing properly. **Don't smack him and only hang him upside down if he's not breathing.** If he doesn't breathe within 30 seconds you can grip him firmly by the ankles, using a towel to prevent slipping and hang him upside down (**c**). Should breathing fail to start, do **gentle** mouth to mouth respiration as described on page 22, **but only 'blow' as much air as you can hold in your cheeks or you'll damage his lungs** (**d**).

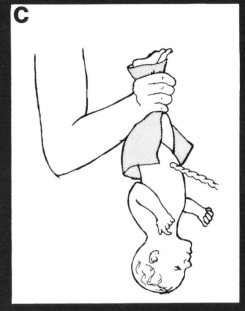

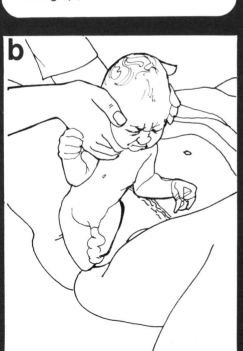

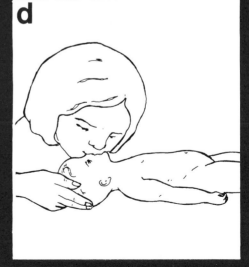

9b Wrap the baby in a warm, soft towel and give him to the mother to hold and put to the breast if the cord is long enough. She will have further contractions and will push the afterbirth out. This can take up to 30 minutes. If you feel confident to cut and tie the cord, do so, but if not, don't worry, provided medical help is on the way. The baby can be left with the mother or in its cot with the cord and afterbirth still attached for a while but keep the afterbirth higher than the baby.

10 Always keep the afterbirth for the doctor or midwife to examine.

11a If you decide to cut the cord, tie one of the pieces of sterilised string very firmly 15cm (6") away from the baby's body and another one a further 5cm (2") away. Cut the cord between the two ties. If the cord end won't stop bleeding, tie another piece of string at about 8–10cm (3–4") away from the baby's body. Keep an eye on the cut end to see that it doesn't bleed. Once the cord is cut, you may find it easier to use elastic bands rather than string.

a

12 Look to see if the birth canal was torn by the baby. If there is severe bleeding even after wiping, press firmly over the area with a pad of clean, freshly laundered nappies, handkerchiefs or a sanitary towel and get medical help.

13 If there are no such complications, reassure the mother that all is well, clean her up as much as possible, put a sanitary towel in place and get her food and drink if she wants some.

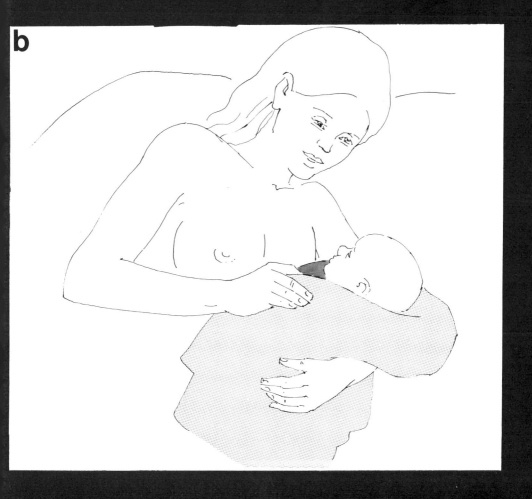

Before you go

Holidays should be a time for the family to enjoy themselves but all too often they are spoilt because of thoughtlessness or ignorance. Most of us go on holiday to do something different from our daily routine and this is the danger because although we're well aware of the hazards around us at home and have learned to live with them, holidays can present entirely new problems.

The most important preparation from the accident point of view is to be well covered by insurance. Illness and accident can strike abroad just as easily as at home but outside the umbrella of the National Health Service the British traveller can find himself in expensive trouble very easily. The European Economic Community provides reciprocal medical cover for people within the Community but outside it bills can mount up very quickly. In order to avail yourself of this though you'll need to have obtained a form E111 from your local DHSS office because without it you'll be treated and have to pay your bills in the foreign country yet may have difficulty claiming the money back. Many holiday companies can arrange insurance as can motoring organisations. You can, of course, also talk to a broker as for any other insurance. Many insurance policies have some provision for the payments involved in bringing back a body in the event of death abroad. Most tour operators offer cover for a sum which is much too small, so it's wise to take extra cover. Multiply your tour operator's figure by 3 to be on the safe side.

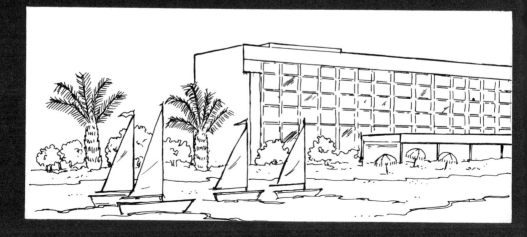

Immunisations

(A useful booklet about these is *Protect your health abroad*, published by the Department of Health & Social Security).

Many countries have immunisation requirements which have to be met before they'll let you in. The diseases that you're most likely to have to be protected against are tetanus, polio, typhoid and yellow fever. Smallpox vaccination is required by fewer and fewer countries as the disease has been eradicated worldwide. It is always difficult to know exactly which immunisations you should have for any given country especially as the regulations sometimes change. Any IATA accredited travel agent (which is most of the reputable ones) can consult a master list he has to tell you exactly what's required or you can phone your airline or the embassy of the country to which you are going. If you are pregnant, have a baby or suffer from a skin complaint, see your doctor for advice about immunisations. Allow yourself a good month to make any health arrangements before going away. Last minute immunisations will not give you such effective protection and may spoil your holiday with a reaction.

Illnesses abroad

The most common illness suffered by holidaymakers is diarrhoea and vomiting. This comes about by consuming food and drink contaminated with food poisoning bacteria and their toxic products. In this country we are very complacent about such bacterial infections because we have drinkable water and the climate doesn't favour rapid bacterial growth in foods. Most of these infections are simply 'holiday tummy' but you can also get more serious conditions such as dysentery or cholera.

To be safe:

1 Boil all drinking water (or use purifying tablets). It's a good idea even to use boiled water for cleaning your teeth.

2 Boil all milk.

3 Peel fresh fruit and avoid salads. Don't just wash fruit and vegetables under water and then eat them. Use cooled, boiled water to clean vegetables.

4 Keep fresh or cooked food in a refrigerator.

5 Drink mineral water or wine if you are unsure of the water and cannot boil it. Even with all these precautions you may still get diarrhoea simply because of the change of food or because your bowel hasn't got used to the new, quite harmless bacteria that inhabit the bowel when you eat and drink in another country.

6 Wash your hands before eating anything.

It's probably a good idea to take an anti-diarrhoea medicine with you because it'll cost a lot more abroad.

Malaria, often thought of as an exotic tropical disease, is being caught by increasing numbers of holidaymakers as package tours venture further afield. It is a very serious disease and can kill you. As there is no vaccination against malaria, you have to cover yourself by taking anti-malaria tablets, even if you are only passing through an infected area. One mosquito bite is all it takes to get the disease. Anti-malaria tablets are available from chemists' shops and airport chemists. You have to take the tablets before you go and keep taking them for six weeks after you return. If you are visiting any of the areas marked on the map, ask your doctor or pharmacist about protection against malaria.

If you should get any illness at all after your return from holiday, tell your doctor at once where you have been and what health precautions you took before and while you were there.

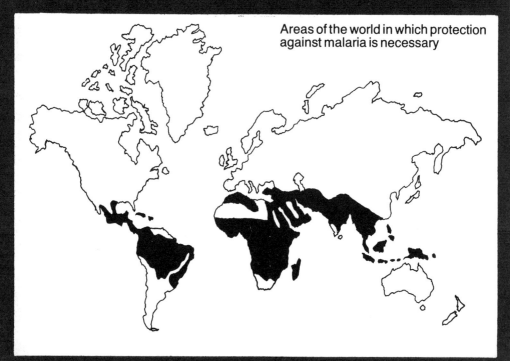

Areas of the world in which protection against malaria is necessary

Travel problems

For details of motion sickness and how to cope with it see page 100. Before taking travel sickness pills, **don't forget to tell your doctor or pharmacist if you are taking any other pills.**

Most of us go on holiday abroad in an aircraft. A short plane journey presents no health problems at all but a longer one can produce ill effects that may mar the start of your holiday.

Here are some tips for long air trips:

1 Drink plenty of non-alcoholic fluid before and during your flight. The air conditioning in the aircraft is very dehydrating and this as much as anything else is what makes people feel bad after a long flight.

2 Get some good sleep before you go as this helps minimise the effect of jet lag.

3 Take things to freshen up in your cabin baggage—you'll feel a lot better when you arrive.

4 Don't overeat or overdrink (alcohol) or you'll pay for it for the next couple of days.

5 Don't plan to do anything too strenuous (if you can arrange this) for the first couple of days after you arrive at your destination. Give your body a chance to get back its balance in the new time zone. Because this can take two days off each end of your holiday it makes sense to travel long distances only for long holidays. It's probably not sensible to go half-way round the world for less than two weeks.

Heat and sun problems

Most of us want sun when we go away but we are unused to it in this country and so may have problems.

There are two types of abnormal reaction to heat—heatstroke and heat exhaustion.

Heatstroke

This happens when the body cannot lose heat, for example in extremely hot climates in which the air is hotter than the body so that the body doesn't lose any heat to the air. It can also occur in very humid conditions which don't allow the body to sweat.

The signs are:

1 Hot, dry, red skin.

2 Rapid pulse.

3 High temperature.

4 Vomiting.

5 Irritability and eventually coma.

Fortunately, this type of heat reaction is uncommon but can be very severe when it does occur and can be dangerous if not treated at once. It comes on rapidly and needs immediate treatment.

What to do:

1 Cool the person by removing his clothes.

2 Fan with an electric fan if you have one.

3 Sponge with tepid water.

4 Call the doctor.

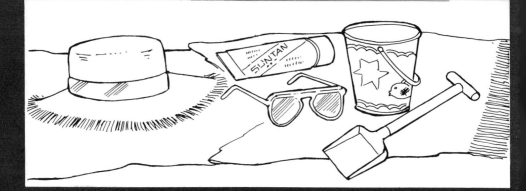

Heat exhaustion
A type of heat problem that comes on slowly and can occur even in this country. It occurs after exceptionally heavy exercise which adds body heat to that from the already hot conditions and it is caused by the body losing too much salt in the sweat. The trouble is thus due to a loss of body salt and water.
The signs are:
1 Normal or slightly raised temperature.
2 Pale, moist skin.
3 Fast, weak pulse.
4 Lethargy, giddiness and headache.
5 Possibly nausea and vomiting.

What to do:
1 Get the person to rest.
2 Give him plenty to drink.
3 Add extra salt to foods and drink as he wants it (half a teaspoonful of salt to one pint of water for an adult).

Prickly heat
An itching skin condition caused by heavy sweating (usually in hot climates). Little red pimples caused by inflammation of sweat ducts occur in the sweaty areas.
What to do:
1 Reduce physical activity (and hence sweating).
2 Don't drink hot drinks.
3 Wear as few clothes as possible (preferably made of a light, natural fibre).
4 Shower in tepid water and use no soap. Dry carefully and use a dusting powder.
5 Soothe bad areas with calamine lotion.
Sunburn
Many a holiday has been spoiled by too much sun too soon. Here are some guidelines:
1 It takes several days to get acclimatised to a sunny climate, so start slowly.

2 Drink plenty of fluids (except alcohol).
3 Only expose yourself for 15–30 minutes for the first day or two.
4 Step this up gradually until by the end of the week you can be out as much as you want. This process takes longer if you are a blonde or a redhead.
5 Use an effective sunscreen lotion or cream.
6 Remember that salty sea water will make you burn faster.
7 When on the water (on a boat, floatable bed etc) remember that the sun is reflected back from the water and that you can get burnt very quickly.
8 Take special care of children as they burn quickly and babies can get heatstroke even by playing on a beach (very reflective and therefore overheating). Make little children wear a hat for the first few days.
9 Wear a hat to keep the sun off your head when you go sightseeing. The time passes quickly when you're absorbed in what you're seeing and you can easily become very hot and burned.
10 Should you get burned, simply apply a cooling lotion (calamine is best).
11 Keep the part covered for a few days.
12 Avoid the strong midday sun—be guided by what the locals do, they know best. if you try to rush getting a tan you'll end up worse off because the sun will knock you out of action for a day or two or you'll be so burned that it will all peel off.

The dangers of water

Whether you are near a pool, boating on a lake, cruising down a canal or sailing on the sea, water is a real hazard that demands great respect.
When at the seaside:
1 Don't bathe when red or other warning flag is up. It's not clever and could endanger someone else's life as he tries to save you.
2 Keep a close eye on children—never let them play at the water's edge unattended. A baby or small child can drown in a few centimetres of water before you even know he's in trouble.
3 Ensure that non-swimmers and all children wear approved and properly constructed life jackets if they are on the water.
4 Look before you dive—many people are seriously ill today because they have hit their heads on rocks or dived into inches of water.
5 If you're on the water either in a boat or water skiing, watch out for bathers. Keep well out of the way or fun can turn to tragedy within a few seconds.
6 For how to treat cramps on or in the water see page 114.
7 Beware of poisonous jellyfish. Most jellyfish are harmless but the Portuguese man-of-war (distinguished by its air-filled bladder that stands up like a sail) is poisonous. Never swim behind a Portuguese man-of-war because the tentacles can stretch up to 45m (50 yards) and bear poisonous capsules. For what to do if stung see page 117.

Listen to the locals when swimming anywhere unfamiliar. With holidays taking people into tropical and sub-tropical waters today many are getting bitten by poisonous fish. Some of these can be dangerous, so ask if it's safe first.

Drowning

Should someone be in trouble in the water either perform proper life-saving techniques if you know how or drag him to shallow water. If he is having great difficulty in breathing (not simply choking, in which case he'll probably clear his own airway adequately), or has stopped breathing:

Don't worry about emptying water out of the lungs—even in someone who has drowned, there is remarkably little water actually in the lungs.

Don't wait until you get to dry land—start mouth to mouth resuscitation (see page 20) at once, as soon as you have a foot on the bottom or can hold on to a boat, for example.

1 Go on with mouth to mouth resuscitation for 1 hour if he doesn't revive before—drowned people can be revived after a much longer time than most people who have stopped breathing.
2 When breathing restarts, put the person into the recovery position (see page 79) with a slight head-down tip.
3 Get him to hospital once breathing is normal.

Climbing, walking and winter sports

The secret of success in these holiday pursuits is careful preparation. The right equipment and clothes can not only improve the pleasure you'll get but may also save your life.

Climbing and walking

1 Make sure you have a large-scale map of the area and be sure that you know how to use it. You'll also need a compass.
2 Take some signalling gear (a whistle and a torch).
3 Take spare socks, a pullover and headgear in case your original ones get wet.
4 Take a simple first aid kit and include crêpe supportive bandages in case of sprains.
5 Take emergency rations, including chocolate and a hot drink in a Thermos flask.
6 Never go off on your own unless you are extremely familiar with the terrain.
7 Let others know where you are going and when you expect to be back or arrive at your destination.
8 Carry a metal foil rescue blanket.
9 Listen to the locals and heed their advice.

The greatest hazard on climbing and walking holidays is exposure. Wetness and wind cool the body and sap the energy of even the fittest people. Eventually, body temperature may sink below normal, with serious consequences or even death.

Signs:
1 Mental and physical slowing.
2 Stumbling and falling.
3 Muscle cramps.
4 Character changes.

Action:
1 Find shelter from the rain or wind.
2 Change into dry clothes if you have them.
3 Keep your head, neck and wrists covered all the time as these areas lose a lot of heat.
4 Drink hot drinks if you have them.
5 Don't wander around wasting valuable body energy—stay put.
6 Erect some kind of signal (eg a highly coloured piece of clothing or rucksack) so that rescuers can find you.
7 When rescuers get within hailing distance, use the International Alpine Distress Signal: six blasts on the whistle, six shouts or six torch flashes. Repeat these at one minute intervals. If no help seems forthcoming, two people should go together for help.
8 Once you get an exposed person to safety, heat him in a warm (not hot) bath, **provided he is conscious.** If he is unconscious from a seriously low body temperature, warm him slowly.
NOTE: People suffering from exposure should be kept flat.

Winter sports
1 Get physically fit before you go as this will reduce the likelihood of injury. Practice skiing on a dry run in this country if you are inexperienced.
2 Buy good protective clothing, always wearing at least two insulating layers beneath your outer ski suit.
3 Don't be fooled by sunshine into forgetting that the temperatures may be below zero. Also protect your skin from sunburn if you're going somewhere sunny.
4 Don't forget that you're very high up and may suffer from altitude sickness. If you feel ill or 'woozy', stay at a lower altitude or don't ski at all for 24 hours.
5 Stay with your party or class—don't wander off unless you are very experienced.
As with sunny holidays—take it easy the first few days. If you're stiff from the unaccustomed exertion you'll be a danger to yourself and others. Much of this can be avoided by careful physical preparation.
6 Make sure you're well insured in case of accident and that the policy covers the cost of bringing you home on a stretcher or in a wheelchair.
7 Always listen to the experts and the locals—they know best.

Although you can always make do in an emergency, it's sensible to have a first aid kit at home. This should be kept in a metal or plastic box, well sealed, and should be stored in a place that doesn't get too steamy. Kitchens and bathrooms are not good places to keep your first aid kit. If you have a first aid kit in the car, don't be put off getting one for the home too. Make sure everyone in the house knows where the first aid kit is and ensure that it stays in the right place. Replace anything you use as soon as possible and keep it away from children.

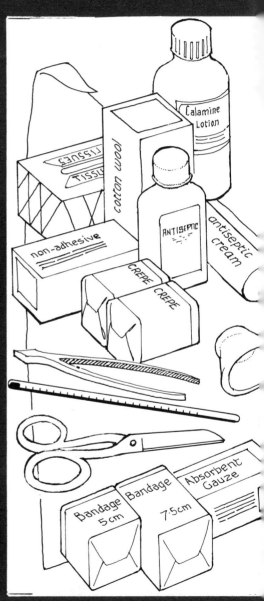

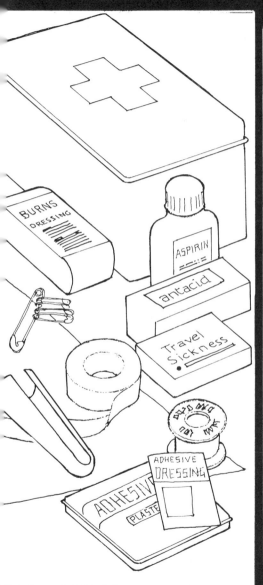

The box should contain:

1 A triangular bandage and several large safety pins.

2 Cotton wool (for cleaning but not for putting on wounds or burns).

3 White gauze in rolls and/or pads.

4 Paper tissues (white preferably) in small unopened packs.

5 Gauze bandages (one 5cm (2in) and one 7.5cm (3in) wide).

6 Crêpe bandages (two of these for putting round bulky dressings or for applying pressure over a pad of gauze on a severely bleeding area. Beware of applying too tightly.

7 Some small sizes of tubular gauze bandage—useful for fingers (the packs have an applicator).

8 Absorbent, non-adhesive dressings. These have gauze on one side and plastic film on the other. The shiny side of the film is placed over the wound and does not stick. The dressings are held in place with a light bandage.

9 Adhesive dressings (plasters) of various sizes.

10 A pre-packed burns dressing.

11 Adhesive strapping.

12 Tweezers for removing splinters.

13 Scissors for cutting bandages and other dressings.

14 Pain-relieving tablets (soluble aspirin or paracetamol). NB. Don't keep aspirin unless foil wrapped for more than a year.

15 Antiseptic for cleaning wounds. It's wise to have both liquid for dilution and some cream to put on the skin direct.

16 Thermometer.

17 Calamine lotion.

18 Indigestion tablets.

19 Travel sickness tablets.

20 An eye bath.

21 Inside the lid of the box write your GP's name and telephone number, also the address and telephone number of the local accident department of your hospital.

What are bandages?

Bandages are strips of material used to support or bind up injured parts of the body. They are made from linen, crêpe, gauze or elasticated material but if you haven't any of these at home, anything will do in an emergency. You could tear up an old pillowcase, sheet or other clean material and use it. Although most bandages are used in strips, a useful bandage is a linen triangular one. It also doubles as a sling.

Bandages are used for:

1 Keeping dressings in place.
2 Giving support to an injured part of the body.
3 Applying pressure over a dressing to stop bleeding.

What are dressings?

Dressings are sterile gauze, lint or cotton wool pads placed directly on a wound, often held in place by a bandage. Increasingly, dressings are either self-adhesive or held in position by adhesive strips. A dressing keeps a wound clean, absorbs blood and other exuded fluids and provides a surface on which antiseptic creams or powders can be placed.

(a) Applying a tubular bandage.
(b) Bandaging an arm.
(c) A wider bandage on the leg.
(d) Using a sling.
(e) Bandaging a hand.

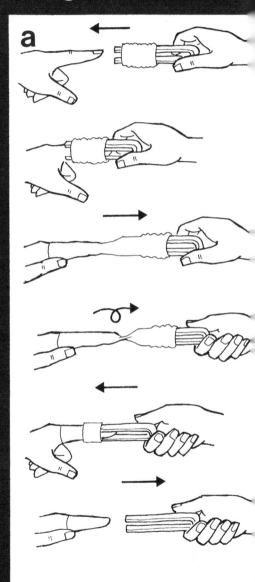

a

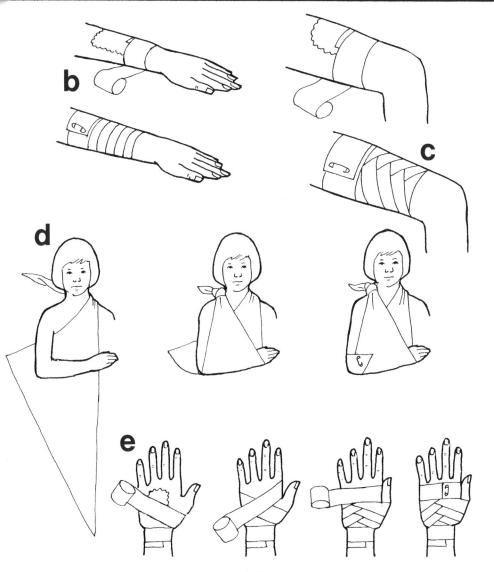

Dressings are used for:

1 Stopping bleeding.
2 Soaking up blood and other body fluids.
3 Keeping germs out of the wound.

They should always be at least clean, preferably sterile and used fresh from a pack. In the absence of a proper dressing, use a clean, freshly laundered handkerchief. There really is no mystery about bandaging and dressing a wound.
Follow these basic principles and you won't go far wrong.

1 Ensure that the worst bleeding is over before applying a dressing (unless you're going to bandage a dressing to stem the flow of blood).
2 If blood comes through one layer of dressing and bandage, apply another layer of each on top of the existing one.
3 Always use a dressing that is plenty big enough.
4 Never apply adhesive dressings close to a wound in such a way that removing the dressing will re-open the wound.
5 Always use a bandage of a width best suited to the area in question. **(a)** On

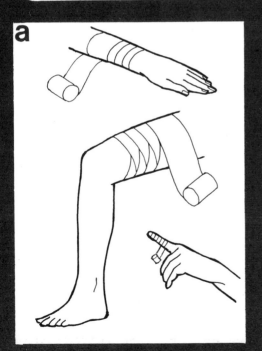

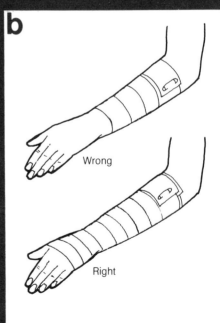

Wrong

Right

the finger, a 2.5cm (1″) bandage is best but for the arm, a 10cm (4″) one is more suitable and for a thigh, a 15cm (6″) one.

6 (c) Hold the rolled-up bandage in your right hand (if you're right handed) and roll the bandage from the inside to the outside of the limb you're bandaging.

7 When applying a bandage, you'll find it easiest to start at the narrowest part of the limb and work towards the widest.

8 Apply the bandage firmly and then secure the end with a safety pin or special bandage clip if you have one.

9 If the person complains of any strange sensations in the part of the limb beyond your bandage, undo it and reapply less tightly. This applies especially for elastic bandages.

10 Always overlap a bandage by about half its width and overlap even more with elastic and crêpe bandages. **(b)** Never leave skin pouting out between the rings of bandage.

11 Remember you are not running a hospital—no one expects you to put on a bandage that will stay there for a week. Simply do the best you can and then get medical help, if necessary.

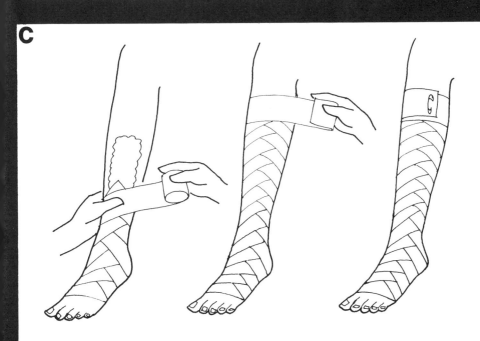

C

How do you know?

1 Breathing stopped:
Check by putting your cheek against the person's mouth or by seeing if a mirror steams up **(a)**.

2 Heartbeat stopped:
Feel the pulse at the neck in the groove at the side of the Adam's apple **(b)** or apply your ear to the left side of the chest for the heartbeat.

3 Cold, pale skin.

4 Unconscious:
Simple efforts fail to rouse. Don't smack hard across the face.

5 Pupils—wide, irregular and motionless.

If the death is expected, don't do heroic life-saving things but respect the dignity of the dead person.

If the death is unexpected, try life-saving procedures. See pages 20 and 24. Call a doctor or ambulance.

If the death is expected, once the doctor has been and given you a certificate:
Don't tie up the chin and remove dentures but if you want to you could remove rings and other valuables from the body before it goes. Be sure to remove wallet, keys etc. You never know when you'll need them.

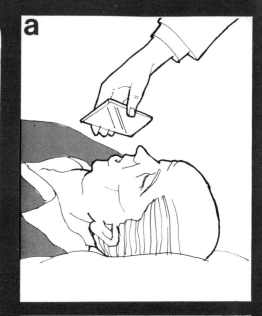

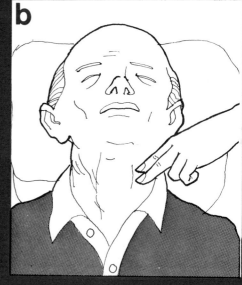

Action:

Depends on whether the death was expected or not.

1 If the person has been suffering from a serious illness or is very old and seems to have died from natural causes, phone his doctor.

2 If the death is unexpected or you suspect suicide, foul play, or an accident, you must phone the police (dial 999). Don't move the body. Don't disturb anything in the room. Stay close by so the police can talk to you.

3 Deaths occurring in an unexpected way will have to be handled by the coroner. The coroner's officer (a policeman) will arrange for the removal of the body. If the dead person hasn't been seen by his doctor within the last 14 days, the coroner is automatically involved and will usually be notified by the doctor.

4 Once the body has been removed, the coroner is responsible for everything until he is satisfied as to the cause of the death. Just because a coroner is involved does **not** mean there will be an inquest. Most coroners' cases are concluded without an inquest. The coroner will probably order a post-mortem for which he does **not** need the consent of the relatives. It is important to know the cause of death in case of any legal proceedings later. It is wise to be represented legally at inquests on deaths resulting from road or industrial accidents as compensation may be payable. Legal aid is not available for coroner's proceedings.

5 Usually death is expected and the person's doctor will decide whether or not he comes himself to see the body. He may simply tell you to ring the undertaker (funeral director) but usually he will come to confirm that the person has died. If you don't know of a funeral director, look in the Yellow Pages. When the doctor comes he will give you a death certificate to take to the Registrar of Births and Deaths.

6 If you are alone in a small house or flat most funeral directors will collect the body and take it to their chapel of rest, even in the middle of the night. This is helpful but can be expensive. Otherwise, wait until office hours and get the funeral director to come in the normal way.

You must register the death by law within 5 days with the Registrar of Births and Deaths. You can get his address and office hours from your local *Citizens Advice Bureau*, town hall, post office, police station, funeral director or telephone book. He will need the death certificate issued by the doctor and, if you have it, the deceased's National Health Service Medical Card.

7 The Registrar will give you a certificate (free of charge) enabling the funeral to take place and also in many cases will issue a special death certificate for National Insurance purposes. If you need certificates as proof of death for insurance companies (to claim life insurance) you must pay for these but the charge is nominal.

Funeral Arrangements

1 If you have been named in the deceased's will as his executor, you will usually make the funeral arrangements.

2 Start on them as soon as you have a death certificate and even before you have been to register the death. If you can't trace a will, don't delay making arrangements.

3 Try to find out whether the deceased wanted to be buried or cremated (this is often in the will). If he is to be cremated, you'll need a special form signed by two doctors.

4 Deal only with a reputable funeral director who is a member of the *National Association of Funeral Directors.*

Always get a written estimate in advance so you know what to expect. Remember—you'll be responsible for the cost of the funeral should there be insufficient money in the estate to cover it. Some funeral directors will want a down payment and some even want all the money before proceeding.

5 Make sure you have a certificate of disposal either from the Registrar of Deaths or the coroner, to give to the funeral director. He cannot actually dispose of the body without it but can start making arrangements.

Benefits payable on death

1 Death Grant. Take the special death certificate from the Registrar to your local social security office. If you cannot go, complete the form on the back of the certificate and send it by post. The death grant stands at £30 but there is talk of raising it.

2 Funeral Grant. A further amount of £30 may be paid if the death of a war pensioner was due to his pensioned disablement.

3 Widow's Benefit. If you are a widow, you may be entitled to certain National Insurance benefits. Ask at your social security office.

4 Supplementary benefit. Anyone who has been left without enough money to live on can claim supplementary benefit. Leaflets and claim forms for this are obtainable at social security offices.

If you have lost a child, the *Compassionate Friends* (see page 112 for address) will be of comfort to you. *Cruse* (see page 112 for address) is an organisation with many local groups that is especially for those who are bereaved.

This book gives you the basic details of self-help and first aid, but there may be occasions when you would like to know more about a particular aspect or application of the subject.

You can learn more on your own from books, which will help you to understand the theory of emergency care, but as the subject is essentially practical, you will learn more from group demonstrations. If you are put off the idea of joining a group because you feel inexperienced and uncertain about the subject, remember that most of the others will be in the same predicament! Also, bear in mind that people interested in first aid are interested in helping others, so patience, compassion and understanding should be among the characteristics of your fellow students and instructors.

Individual learning

This will be mainly by book work, though you may consider volunteering to work in a cottage or bigger hospital casualty department in the evening to learn whilst helping. Obviously a hospital has a limit to the number of people who can assist like this and often the person will be expected to have some first aid experience, but this need not necessarily be the case and untrained people can be of tremendous help to such departments. Don't go expecting drama but rather to give a simple service with the opportunity to learn much about handling the ill and injured.

There are a number of books on the subject of first aid (see page 155). Some are written as handbooks for organised courses of instruction; others are meant for reading on your own; and then there are those designed to consult in a crisis.

Decide what you want out of a book on the subject, consider how best you learn—by words or pictures—and then examine the book in detail. Read the description on the cover, and the preface. The book should tell you for what purpose it has been written and at what level. Look at the illustrations and consider what information they offer you and then choose a subject you know something about—perhaps an injury that someone you know has suffered. Look it up in the index and read the appropriate section. Does it tell you anything new, can you understand it, and do you find the presentation easy to concentrate on? If you are comparing books, make this same subject test on each one to help you find which book is best suited to your requirements. Finally, look at the index. If it is very brief, how are you going to find details in the book, especially in an emergency?

Most of the books in the list on page 155 are relatively inexpensive and have been chosen as having most to offer in their field. Remember that you can borrow a book from the library to examine in more detail before buying a copy to keep for reference.

Group learning

It is a very good idea to have a basic working knowledge of first aid and self help. We live in a mechanised age of rapid travel and high technology and the potential for injury is all around us. Being prepared for the worst is a sound insurance policy. An awareness of potential danger is also probably the best form of safety education as prevention is always better than cure.

Probably the most universally successful and available way to learn more is to join a first aid course organised by the *St John Ambulance Association*, the *British Red Cross Society* or the *St Andrew's Ambulance Association*. You don't have to join the association if you don't want to. Just enrol for a course, which won't be expensive. You can obtain further details from local secretaries (look up the association in the telephone book). A course may extend to several weeks of hourly evening sessions, or be a short 'crash' course. You may become so interested that you decide to join the particular association and go on duty in local theatres, cinemas and sports halls or even drive their ambulances to local gymkhanas and motor scrambles.

Motoring organisations (*A.A.* and *R.A.C.*) sometimes offer short courses in practical first aid—perhaps in combination with a lecture from a police driver on better driving techniques. Local enquiry will enable you to reserve a place on the next course.

If you have an occupational interest in the subject you may be able to suggest that your firm, union, trade association or club organises a course or even a talk or film on a particular aspect of first aid. Many first aid associations, community ambulance services and local doctors organise lectures, demonstrations or films on request.

Audio-visual material

Doctors can hire films from the *Graves' Medical Audio-visual Library* and film strips can be bought from commercial companies such as *Camera Talks*. These are all listed in a catalogue of audiovisual material published by the *St John Ambulance Association Headquarters at 1 Grosvenor Crescent, London SW1*. You may be able to organise meetings in conjunction with a Health and Safety at Work Committee or attend evening classes at local educational establishments. You may want to suggest that your children have the opportunity to learn more about first aid at school by raising the matter at Parent Teacher Association meetings.

Women's associations such as the *Women's Institute* and *Townswomen's Guild*, or men's associations such as the *Rotary*, the *Round Table* and *Lions Clubs* can request speakers on first aid or related subjects such as crime prevention (local police), fire prevention (local fire station), rescue (coastguards), the lifeboat service (*R.N.L.I.*) and lifesaving (*Royal Lifesaving Society*). *RoSPA (the Royal Society for the Prevention of Accidents)* produce posters and other educational material on the subject. All of these ideas can be used to create interest in first aid through existing clubs and societies.

Other interesting books

Title: The Essentials of First Aid.
Publishers: The St John Ambulance Association.
Date: Revised Edition 1983.
Price: £2.45.

Title: Bailliere's Handbook of First Aid.
Edited by Stanley Miles.
Publishers: Bailliere Tindall.
Date: 6th Revised Edition, July, 1970.
Price: £4.50.

Title: How to Survive.
Author: Brian Hildreth.
Publishers: Puffin Books.
Date: May, 1982.
Price: £1.10.

Title: The First Aid Manual (The official textbook
   of the three first aid organisations).
Publishers: Dorling Kindersley in association with
   The St John Ambulance Association and
   The British Red Cross Society.
Price: £5.95 hardback.
         £3.95 paperback.

Title: Caring for the Sick.
Publishers: Dorling Kindersley in association with
   The St John Ambulance Association and
   The British Red Cross Society.
Price: £5.95 hardback.
         £3.95 paperback.

Advanced First Aid Reading:

Title: New Advanced First Aid.
Authors: A. Ward Gardner and Peter J. Roylance.
Publishers: John Wright.
Date: 2nd Revised Edition, June, 1977.
Price: £4.50.

Title: Diagnosis Before First Aid.
Author: Neville Marsden.
Publishers: Churchill Livingstone.
Date: July, 1978.
Price: £3.25.

156 Glossary

A glossary of terms used in first aid though not necessarily in this book

Abrasion—skin graze.
Airway—major passage for air through nose and mouth to windpipe.
Analgesic—pain-relieving drug.
Antidote—drug given to counteract poison.
Antiseptic—chemical used to kill germs.
Apoplexy—stroke.
Asphyxia—obstructed breathing.

Bacteria—germs.
Blanket lift—use of a blanket to 'cradle-lift' a patient.
Blister—collection of fluid under a thin layer of damaged skin.
Broad bandage—made from folding triangular bandage into broad strip.
Bruise—leakage of blood in or under the skin following injury.
Burn—heat damage to body tissues.

Cardiac massage or compression—hand pressure on breastbone to squeeze the heart rhythmically and maintain circulation.
Closed fracture—broken bone with intact overlying skin.
Cold compress—wet bandage or application to relieve swelling or bruising.
Coma—state of unconsciousness from which person cannot be aroused.
Complicated fracture—broken bone associated with damage to another structure such as a blood vessel or nerve.
Compression bandage—firm, often padded bandage applied to control swelling or bleeding.
Concealed haemorrhage—bleeding internally.
Contusion—wound caused by crushing.
Convulsion—fit.
Crêpe bandage—elasticated bandage that supports and conforms to body contours.
Cyanosis—blueness of skin from shortage of oxygen in the blood.

Diagnosis—opinion of the nature of a complaint or injury—a medical 'label'.
Dislocation—joint out of socket.
Dressing (field)—wound covering often of standard 'pad and bandage' pattern.
Dyspnoea—difficulty with breathing.

Elevation—raising of injured or bleeding limb to reduce swelling or bleeding.
Emetic—drug given by doctor to provoke vomiting.
Epilepsy—a condition in which there are fits or convulsions.
Exhale—breathe out.
Exposure—a condition leading to body chilling and then to an abnormally low body temperature.

Faint—lowering of blood pressure and loss of consciousness due to emotional shock or hot stuffy conditions.
Figure of eight bandage—double encircling bandage (to support foot and ankle, for example).
First aid—immediate treatment carried out before definitive medical care.
Floater bandage—bandage of variable position.
Flushing—reddening of the skin.
Foreign body—substance embedded in a wound, eye or body orifice.
Fracture—break in a bone.
Friction burn—skin burn caused by rubbing or chafing.
Frostbite—skin damage to the extremities from extreme cold.

Gauze dressing—open-weave, non-fluffy material used to cover wounds.

Haematoma—collection of blood in bruised area.
Haemorrhage—bleeding.
Heart massage—see cardiac massage.
Heat exhaustion—weakness from loss of body salt and water.

Heat stroke—rapid collapse with high temperature.
Hypertension—abnormally high blood pressure.
Hypothermia—extreme lowering of body temperature.
Hysteria—extreme emotional over-reaction.

Ice pack—application of ice and water to injury to reduce swelling and pain.
Immobilisation—splinting or firm support of an injury.
Incision—cutting type of wound.
Infection—invasion of body tissues by germs.
Inflatable splint—blow-up plastic envelope limb support.
Inhale—breathe in.

Laceration—jagged wound.
Lint—non-fluffy, close-weave material used for covering wound.
Locked knee—inability to straighten knee.

Morphine—drug used to relieve severe pain.

Open fracture—broken bone with overlying skin wound.

Padding—soft cushioning between or around injuries.
Pallor—pale, blood-drained skin.
Paralysis—loss of ability to control muscle movements.
Plaster of Paris—bandage impregnated with gypsum which sets hard after being dipped in water.
Pressure bandage—firm bandage used to control severe bleeding.
Pressure points—areas where hand or finger pressure will compress an artery to reduce drastic bleeding (rarely used).
Prone—lying face down.
Pulse—pressure wave of heart pump action that can be felt over arteries (usually at wrist and neck).
Puncture wound—wound caused by pointed object penetrating skin.

Pus—fluid consisting mostly of white blood cells that have been involved in fighting invasion of germs.
Recovery position—a vital position to prevent choking in an unconscious patient—see page 78.
Respiration—breathing.
Resuscitation—revival of patient.

Scald—skin damage from hot liquid or steam.
Seat lift—lifting a patient by interlocked hand/wrist grip.
Shock—severe bodily reaction to injury.
Signs—visible or detectable evidence of patient's illness or injury.
Sling—triangular shaped material used for supporting an arm.
Spasm—involuntary contraction of muscle.
Splint—firm support used to immobilise an injured area.
Sprain—damage to the ligament around a joint, often with blood loss into the area.
Stab wound—wound caused by sharp puncture of skin.
Strain—damage to a muscle.
Stretcher—device for carrying a patient in the horizontal position.
Stupor—degree of unconsciousness.
Sucking wound—chest wound with drawing of air into wound.
Supine—lying on the back.
Symptoms—things a person complains of—evidence of his illness or injury.
Syncope—faint.

Tendon—sinew, leader.
Thrombosis—clotting of blood.
Tourniquet—constricting bandage or band applied to stop passage of blood through arteries and veins. Not to be used by the inexperienced.
Traction—application of hand or mechanical pulling to control a fracture.
Triangular bandage—triangular-shaped material used for making sling or other support.

Varicose veins—distended visible veins, usually in leg.

Main references are in heavy type.